HOW TO
LOOK GOOD
NAKED
CAN CHANGE YOUR LIFE

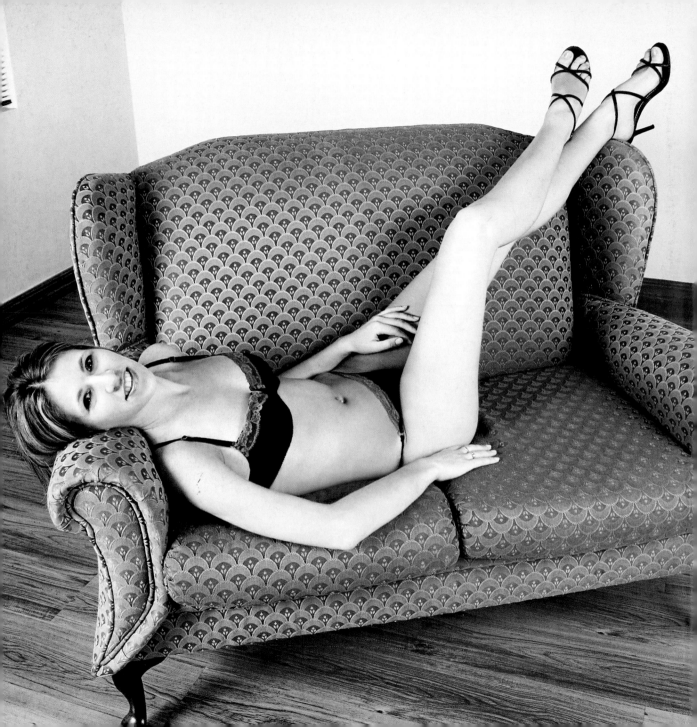

HOW TO
LOOK GOOD
NAKED

CAN CHANGE YOUR LIFE

Charmaine Yabsley

A Cassell Book
An Hachette Livre UK Company

First published in the UK 2009 by Cassell Illustrated,
a division of Octopus Publishing Group Ltd.
2–4 Heron Quays,
London E14 4JP

A CIP catalogue record for this book is available from the British Library.

ISBN-13: 978-1-84403-677-6

10 9 8 7 6 5 4 3 2 1

Commissioning Editor: Laura Price
Cover artwork: Lee Binding
Design and text: Essential Works
Production: Caroline Alberti

Printed in China

Contents

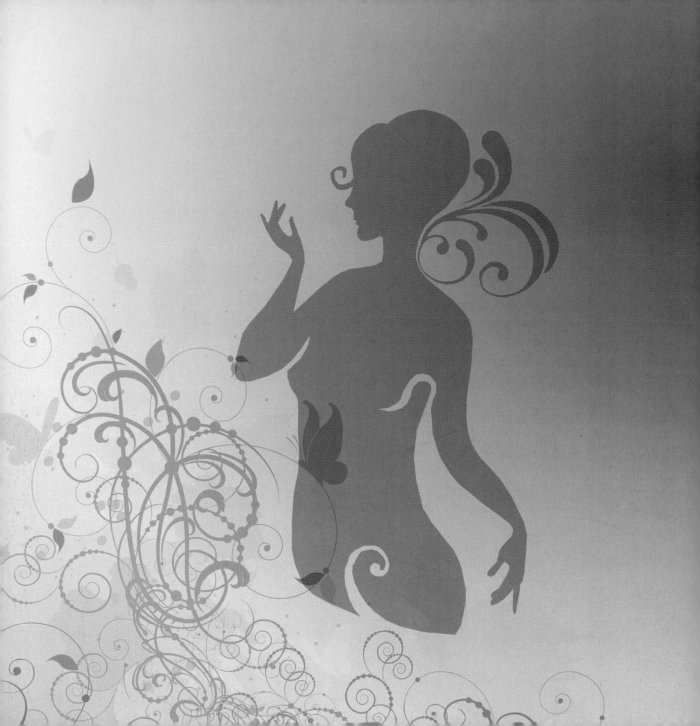

Chapter 1

OUR BODIES AND US

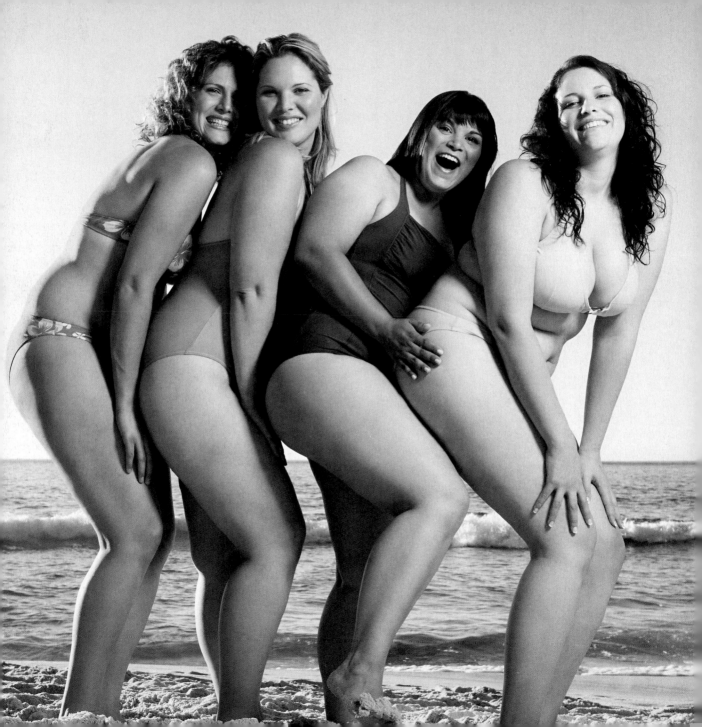

Girls of Great Britain! It's time to stop body loathing and start body loving. Whether you're big, small, tall or short you're all gorgeous lovelies who need the confidence to get out of your big baggy clothes and into some seriously sexy outfits.

So what's holding you back from being the best you can be? We know that around 90% of you dislike your body, with a massive 75% of you obsessing over a particular body part throughout the day. This is serious. You need to leave your body hang-ups behind and let it all hang out.

The key is to understand your body shape – and this is what this book is all about. We identify the 'Rules' for dressing your particular silhouette, as well as giving you great 'Salon style' beauty advice to get you gorgeous from head to toe – so that you look just as good naked as you do dressed. And once you know how to dress for your shape then there's nothing to stop you from looking absolutely fabulous 24-7.

And remember, looking fabulous isn't just about wearing the right jacket or heels (although that helps!). Looking fantastic is all about feeling and acting confident. So pull those shoulders back, hold your heads up high, and get ready to look good naked!

SOME STATISTICS

- 81% of women in the UK are ashamed of how they look
- A whopping 90% aren't comfortable about being naked in front of their friends
- 78% have stretch marks
- 97% of women wish they had longer legs
- 87.5% of women want to be taller
- 60% of women are pear-shaped
- 31% are pencil-shaped
- Just 6% of women are now hourglass-shaped

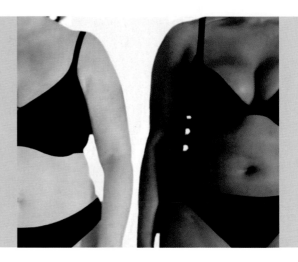

In a sense some of the statistics above make depressing reading – will us ladies of Great Britain ever learn how to feel good about our bodies? Yet perhaps at the same time all you women out there who are feeling bad about yourselves can find some reassurance in the fact that you are most certainly, assuredly, not alone.

The passage from acutely negative body image to super confidence doesn't usually happen overnight (although it can!). We hope, though, that you'll find inspiration in the stories of the girls who came on the show and managed to genuinely transform their relationship with their bodies. We hope, too

'Since 1920 the average breast size has increased by 4 inches, hip size by 6 inches and waist size by 8 inches.'

that this book will help you at least some way on your journey to improved self-esteem.

The statistics below tell us about something else that has been happening to our bodies in recent times – it is clear that as a nation we are getting larger. This can largely be explained by a mixture of diet and lifestyle factors. The diet of the early 1950s – despite the hangover of wartime rationing – was significantly healthier than it is today, with meals of meat and two veg being at the heart of family living. Today, by contrast, a lifestyle of less regular mealtimes and takeaway meals, which are full of added sugar, salt and preservatives, coupled with a more inactive, sofa-bound lifestyle, has led to an inevitable expansion in our bums and waistlines.

We now exercise less than three times a week, whereas 50 years ago a sedentary lifestyle was seen as the preserve of the upper classes only. Most ordinary people would walk, ride or do some form of heart-pumping activity for at least two hours a day. It's no wonder we've ballooned. In fact, while there is seemingly no escape from the super-skinny celebrity, constantly forced upon us by glossy magazines, this image bears less and less resemblance to the woman on the street.

Wouldn't life be so much easier if we could just accept ourselves as we are?

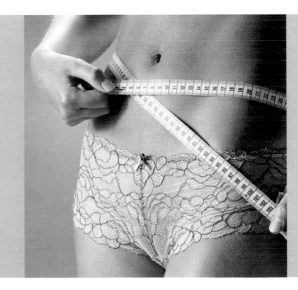

- Since 1920 the average UK breast size has increased by 4 inches, hip size by 6 inches and waist size by 8 inches.
- In the last 50 years the average woman has grown by an inch, to 5 feet 4 inches.
- During the past 80 years our feet have increased from a size 4 to a size 6.
- The average woman now has a 36.5-inch bust, a 30-inch waist and 39.5-inch hips. In 1920 these vital statistics were 32 inches, 22 inches and 33.5 inches respectively.
- The average bra cup size has gone from a B to a C.

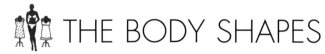

THE BODY SHAPES

Apple, Pear, Pencil? Which body shape are you? We all come in different shapes and sizes: some of us are tall and thin, others short and shapely. Knowing your shape is the first step in finding out how to make the most of your body. There are six basic body shapes, and they are described below. Once you know what to accentuate and what to camouflage you can hit the high street with confidence. And best of all, with the right clothing know-how you'll even be able to turn an apple into an hourglass or a petite princess into a leggy lovely.

YOU'RE AN APPLE BODY SHAPE IF:

- your hips and bum are slightly smaller in width than your chest and tummy;
- you have a rounded tummy;
- your arms are slim and long;
- you have well-shaped, slender legs;
- you have large boobs.

AT-A-GLANCE CLOTHING GUIDE – APPLE

- Leggings and skinny jeans streamline your legs and, teamed with a loose fitting A-line or trapeze dress, trick the eye into thinking your entire body is long and thin.
- High-waisted pencil skirts with big wide belts hold you in and give you an hourglass waist.
- Short, loose dresses or tunics show off your legs and arms while concealing your stomach.
- A-line or swing coats are a great way to look shapely and stylish in cold weather.
- Strappy high heels make your lovely legs look even leggier.

YOU'RE A PEAR BODY SHAPE IF:

- you have small, pert breasts;
- you have a long waist;
- you have a flattish tummy;
- your shoulders are narrower than your hips;
- you're a size larger on the bottom than you are on top;
- you have largish thighs and shortish legs.

AT-A-GLANCE CLOTHING GUIDE – PEAR

- Bootcut jeans and trousers will balance out your hips and thighs.
- Straight-leg, high-waisted trousers elongate your bottom half. Look for lengths that hit the floor and team with heels for a sexy, powerful shape.
- Dresses with a belt accentuate your waist. Structured shift dresses highlight your waist whilst gently skimming your hips and bum.
- Hats take attention away from your hips. A beret adds a shot of Parisian chic, whereas a funky trilby is a cheeky 'look-at-me' accessory.

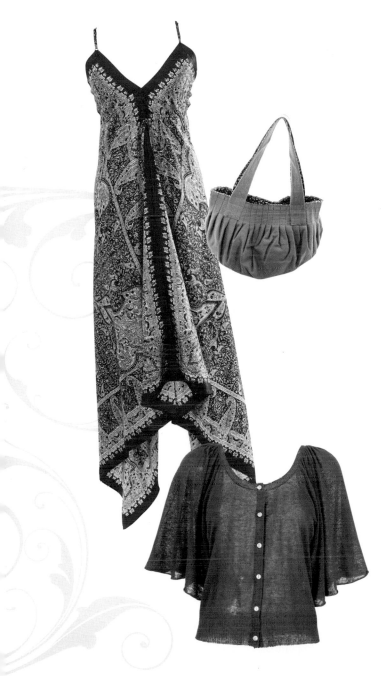

YOU'RE AN HOURGLASS BODY SHAPE IF:

- your boobs are the same measurement as your hips;
- your waist is much smaller than your hips;
- you have shapely, broad shoulders;
- you have shapely legs that end with neat little ankles;
- your silhouette is similar to a figure of 8.

AT-A-GLANCE CLOTHING GUIDE – HOURGLASS

- Dark denim will slim down your hips and bum. The darker your jeans or trousers the smaller you'll seem. Big back pockets will make your bum look even smaller.
- A V-neck will elongate your neck, perk up your boobs and show off your cleavage
- Fitted waistcoats will emphasize your waist.
- Height will always flatter your figure so heels are great for you.
- Pull your hair into a ponytail and accessorize with big dangly earrings to highlight your shoulders.
- Belts with every outfit will highlight your tiny waist.

YOU'RE A PENCIL BODY SHAPE IF:

- you have similar measurements for your boobs, waist and hips;
- your legs are longer than your torso;
- your legs and arms tend to be slender;
- you have an athletic or boyish figure.

AT-A-GLANCE CLOTHING GUIDE – PENCIL

- Bright shift dresses highlight your slender frame. Try necklines that widen your upper half, as this will shrink your hips and bottom.
- Belts transform your pencil into an hourglass.
- Dresses that cling to every curve give great shape. A little cardigan or jacket adds oomph up top.
- Structured jackets, shirts and coats that nip in at the waist are great for you.
- Brightly-coloured tops with slim black trousers give you endless legs and a curvy top half.

YOU'RE A TALL AND LONG BODY SHAPE IF:

- you're more than 5ft 8in;
- you have long slender legs and a long upper body;
- your arms are long and slim;
- your shoulders are narrow.

AT-A-GLANCE CLOTHING GUIDE – TALL AND LONG

- A maxi dress is the ultimate style for the tall and long girl. Wear a bright colour and flaunt your sexy shoulders.
- A belted funnel-neck coat with a waist-cinching belt gives gorgeous curves. A frill-edge coat adds femininity.
- Knee-length boots give shape to your calves.

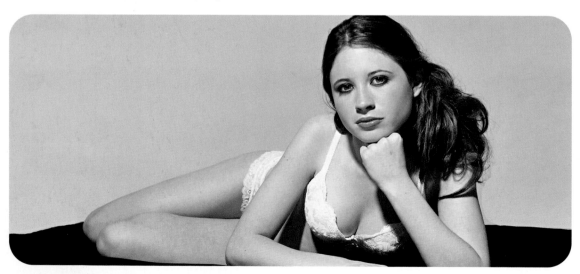

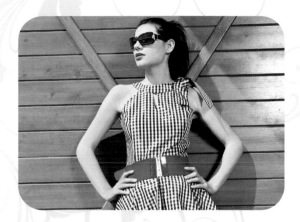

YOU'RE A PETITE BODY SHAPE IF:

- you're 5ft 3in or under;
- you have short legs;
- you have a short torso;
- you have a slim waist;
- you have narrow hips.

AT-A-GLANCE CLOTHING GUIDE – PETITE

- Dresses in simple shapes and bold colours make you appear taller. Pile your hair up high and get into hats.
- High-waisted flares give you the illusion of longer legs. With denim, go for a snug fit as baggy jeans can drown you.
- Heels are a must. Shoes the same colour as your legs or tights give the illusion of longer legs. Platforms when you're in trousers or jeans are perfect.
- For a really luxurious look go for a satin blouse and pencil skirt, some heels and fishnets!

- A long skinny scarf encourages the eye to move up and down your body, and tricks it into thinking you are taller.

It is possible to be a mixture of two shapes, most typically a pear and an hourglass, but this is usually explained by outside factors such as having had children or your typical diet. For example, you are an hourglass but you've morphed into a bit of an apple because of too many lagers! Your basic shape remains an hourglass, however.

So now you know how to dress your body shape – or at least you will when you've finished reading the pages that follow. But, as we've said, that's not the whole story. Let's face it, even if you've got your dressing code completely sussed, you're not going to turn any heads if your eyes are fixed firmly on the ground and your shoulders are slumped forwards. Confidence is the key to making any outfit look good: if you believe that you're gorgeous, sexy and fabulous then others will too. It really is as simple as that.

Still confused about your shape? Here's a quick way to find out your type. Lie down on a full-length piece of paper and get someone to draw round you. This will help you see the real you and enable you to identify whether you are Apple, Pear, Hourglass, Pencil, Tall and long or Petite.

SEVEN WAYS TO BOOST YOUR CONFIDENCE

1 Stand up straight. The quickest way to look confident – and lose 5lbs – is to pull those shoulders back, hold your head up high, pull your tummy in and tuck your bottom under. Add some eye-catching lippy and smile your sexy smile. You can't fail!

2 Focus on the next five minutes. Stop looking at what you can't do, or don't have. Instead, concentrate on using just the next five minutes to your best ability. Instead of reaching for a cookie for a quick energy fix, drink a glass of water and call a friend for a gossip. Let this five minutes turn into 20 minutes and before you know it you're down mood or urge to pig out will have passed.

3 Get specific about why you want what you want. Many of us say we want to be thinner/fitter/younger-looking etc but you need to ask yourself what do you think being thinner/fitter/younger looking will get you? More respect, more love, more happiness, more freedom? Once you're clear in your mind, record a tape of yourself answering the following questions:

• What will it be like to have more..........(you fill in the blank – freedom/love/happiness) in my life?

• How will I feel when I wake up in the morning/when I go to bed at night?

• How will I handle any future challenges feeling my new feelings?

• What will be different in my life? How will others react to me? What will I look like? How will I feel about myself?

• What advice will I give to others about how they can feel this way too?
Listen to that tape every day. Getting to the root of what you really want in life and then spelling out the actions that will get you more of that is a very motivating strategy.

4 Set yourself up to succeed by under-promising. If your pattern is to promise to drink water, eat rice cakes and run for an hour every day for the next 30 days, it's time you stopped sabotaging your success and got realistic. Set yourself achievable goals and then lower the bar. Under-promise, over-deliver and you'll feel like you're actually gaining something rather than feeling that you are always failing.

5 Celebrate every molehill. Don't wait until you've reached the top of the mountain before you crack open the champagne. Acknowledge your small achievements every day and create a reward system – from allowing yourself a lie-in on Saturday for going for an early morning run in the week to buying flowers for eating healthily for three days in a row.

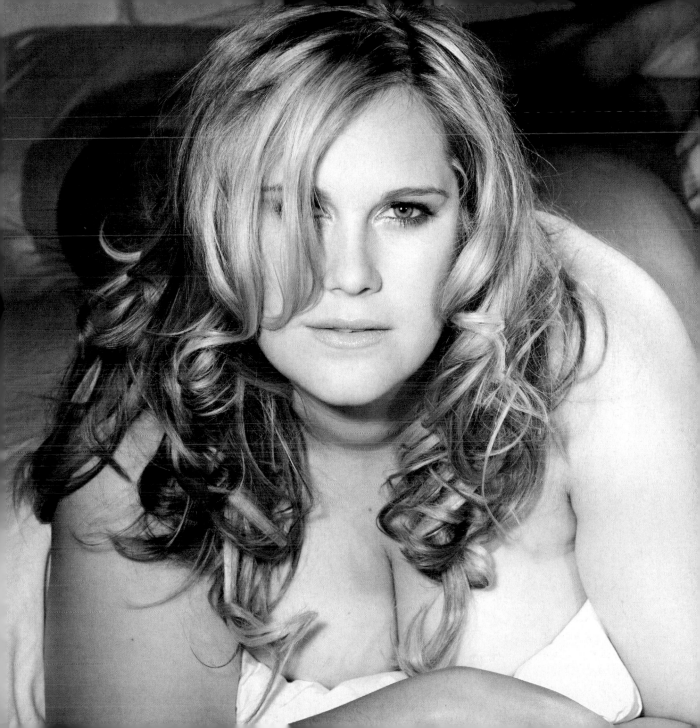

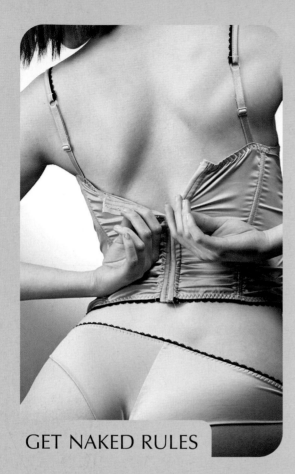

GET NAKED RULES

As we've explained, in the pages that follow you'll learn how to get your body shape and wardrobe into good working order, but that's not where our work stops! After all, the title of this book is How to Look Good Naked. So here are your seven Rules for getting your kit off with confidence. Use this as a checklist – all these salon tricks are expanded upon further in the book.

1 Exfoliate, exfoliate, exfoliate. Yes, we know that you're sick of hearing it, but it's good advice for good reason. It works! Exfoliation not only sloughs off dead skin cells but it also increases your circulation, so your skin will look all glowing and gorgeous.

2 Fake tan. We don't want you to resemble a footballer's wife, but a subtle golden glow will make you look thinner, healthier and camouflage any lumps and bumps. If you don't want to go the full monty with a fake tan, then use a self-tanning moisturizer, which will gradually add a soft glow to your skin.

3 Add some scent. Scented moisturizers are a good way to layer your favourite smell. Then dab some perfume on your erogenous zones: behind your knees, ears and wrists.

4 Add some body-smoothing highlighter (see p.43) – along your collarbone to catch the light, and down your shin, to make your legs appear slimmer.

5 Make sure your manicure and pedicure are up to scratch. Repair any hangnails or chipped polish.

6 Add some high heels – you'll look instantly thinner as you will be forced to stand up straighter. You'll look more confident too.

7 Whether you're a size 0 or a size 20, if you hold your head up high while wearing nothing but a smile you'll look sexy and instantly kissable.

'Celebrate every molehill. Don't wait until you've reached the top of the mountain before you crack open the champagne. Acknowledge your small achievements every day.'

6 Focus on how great you are. Low self-esteem is often at the root of poor motivation because, deep down, we don't think we can change or we don't believe we are good enough to reach our goals. To boost self-esteem, give yourself positive messages about yourself constantly. Write down 10 messages such as 'You are a kind and thoughtful person' to 'You are wise and wonderful' and stick them all round your house/on your bedroom mirror/on the fridge door for seven days. After seven days you usually stop seeing them, so write down another 10 messages. What you focus on expands. That's how you know it's time to change your focus.

7 Change WHO you are as well as WHAT you do. When you change behaviour you usually just change what you're doing. In other words, if you want to be healthier you stop eating cake and start going swimming on Monday. Try a different approach and ask yourself:

WHO do I want to become? (for example, you may think: 'I am someone who takes care of my body at such a luxurious level that I feel pampered.') Ask yourself what actions this this person would take. Alternatively, if you want to be a person who has enormous amounts of energy, think about what you would eat, how you would deal with stress, and how would get up each morning. The focus is on creating a new identity for yourself versus simply trying to change what you are doing. Be patient as it can take a while for the results to show, but if you follow this advice the changes are usually permanent.

Now let's meet the girls…

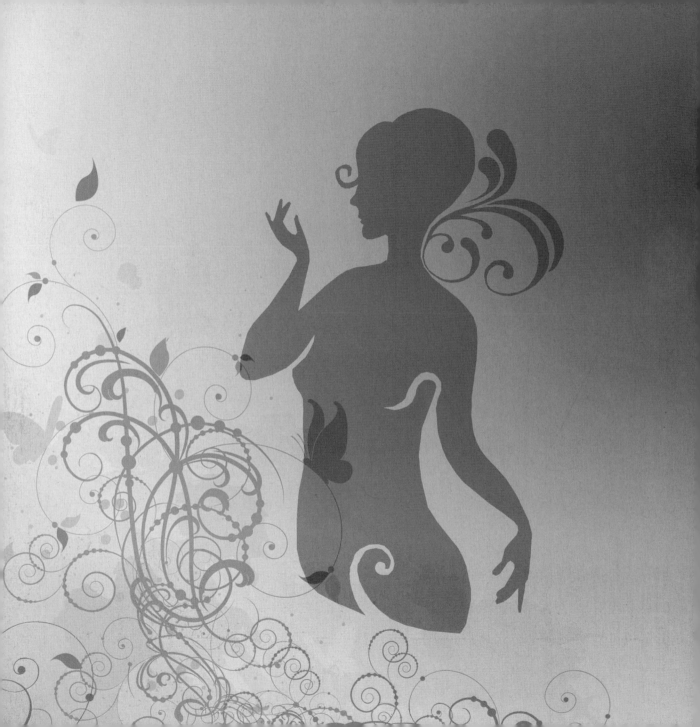

Chapter 2

BUST BLUES

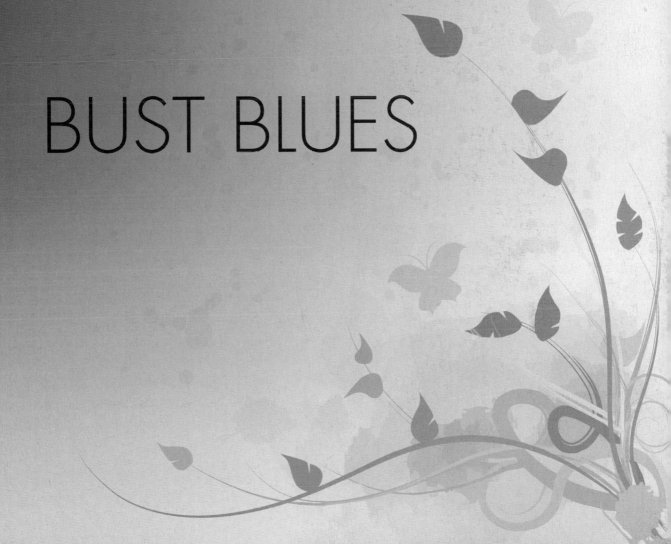

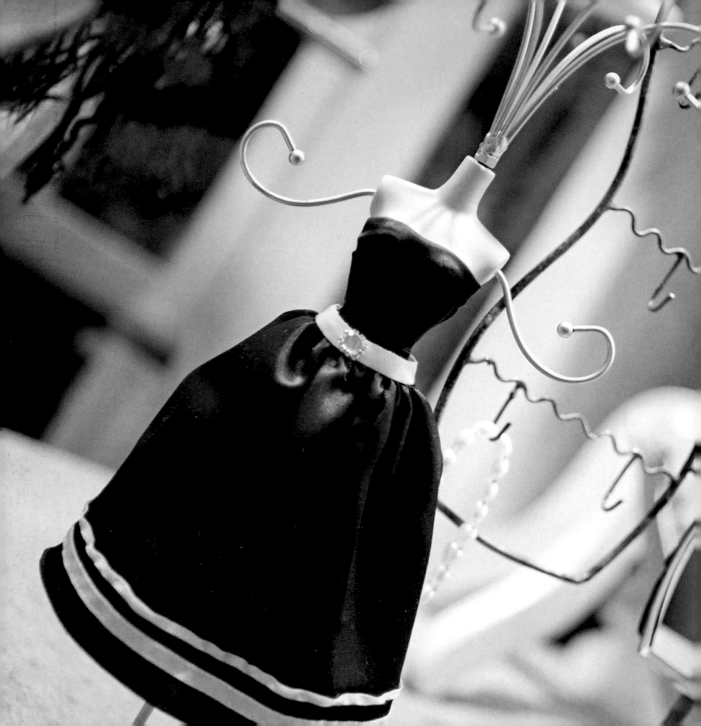

CURVES
OUT OF CONTROL

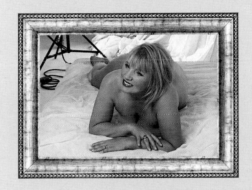

Susan Sharpe, 46, from London's Notting Hill, has a classic hourglass figure: curvy and womanly. Yet like nine out of ten British women, she hated everything about her body. A Yorkshire lass who lived the London life, Susan had curves to die for but kept them securely under wraps. Susan was an average size 16, but felt that her figure was anything but average. She hated her body so much that she hadn't been on a holiday for five years, because she couldn't bear the thought of getting into a swimsuit. And it wasn't only holidaymakers who were denied a peek at Susan's beautiful body – her husband Robert wasn't allowed a look either. Susan went to extremes to make sure Robert never saw her naked, sneaking into bed when he wasn't looking or waiting until he was asleep and the lights were off. Anything to avoid being looked at.

Our mission was to show Susan how to shine the spotlight on her womanly curves and dress her classic shape with fashions that really did it justice. In the process we taught Susan how to go from bad bras and droopy boobs to a body she could really love.

IN THE MIRROR

Susan hadn't been naked in front of anybody for three years. 'All I see when I look at my reflection is a fat woman,' she said. 'It's awful. It's just fat and awful.' We didn't want to tell Susan she had to lose weight or firm up; we wanted to show her instead how to love what she had and to flaunt it. 'You're better when you're thinner and straight up and down, because that's what people see in magazines. I'm not like that, and that's why I've covered myself up,' she said. She saw only flaws: fat, flab and cellulite. Yet when we asked people on the street what they saw when they looked at a picture of Susan in her underwear, there were unanimous votes of admiration for her sexy legs, beautiful breasts and womanly curves.

BODY PERCEPTION

We brought Susan in amongst a group of women who all had fabulous curves. They ranged from a petite 38-in hip measurement to a more generous 47in. We asked Susan – who has 42-inch hips – where she thought she belonged in the line-up. Susan placed herself as the largest of all the women; she believed her hips were more than five-and-a-half inches larger than they really were. Even when we showed Susan just how small her hips were we had trouble convincing her, she was so sure that she belonged at the bigger end of the scale.

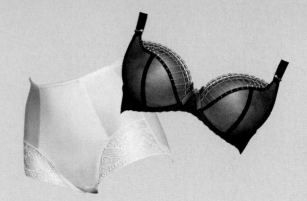

Going undercover

- If you're heavy up top, then give your boobs the support they need. Underwired bras are best: the wire should lie on your chest wall.

- Test the fit by lifting your arms up in the air – if the bra stays put then it's a perfect fit.

- To get your boobs eye-poppingly perfect, choose an underwired bra with no padding.

- The cup should cover the entire breast.

- Even strapless bras can give you support, as long as the size is right.

- If you've got love handles around your waist, choose deep briefs with generous elastic and high-cut legs.

- Avoid sporty shorts – they'll only make your bottom look bigger and your thighs even thicker.

- Make the most of your waist by smoothing the area out – high-cut waists are ideal.

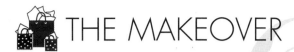

THE MAKEOVER

We showed Susan how to lift those boobs, tone that tum and shape that bum. It's all about dressing your body shape and making the most of what you've got. All gain and no pain. It had been six years since Susan had worn a dress and we needed to remind her what a wonderful woman she was.

Susan was so excited about her makeover. Once she saw what a difference the right sort of clothes made, she was ready to succumb to our beauty treatments for a new top-to-toe look, which included a salt and clay body wrap that helped her lose two inches off her waist and hips (see below).

Salon Style

BODY WRAPS

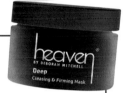

Body wraps work by drawing out toxins and excess water from the body, so they're a great last-minute fix if you need to fit into that little black dress or hit the beach. If you don't have time to get to a salon, you can achieve similar results at home.

Exfoliate your body from top to toe. If you don't have a specially formulated exfoliator, then mix a tablespoon of sugar into your body wash and scrub all over (though you should avoid using this on your face).

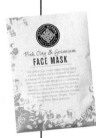

Fill up your bathtub with 250g of Epsom salts. These contain magnesium, which helps eliminate toxins and banish bloating. Soak in the bathtub for at least 20 minutes. While you're soaking, apply a face and hair mask as well.

Once you're sufficiently soaked, get out of the bath and apply a body oil all over your damp skin.

Wear some warmish pyjamas to help keep the detox going. Put some thick moisturizer onto your feet and pop some socks on. This will help moisturize your tootsies while you're sleeping. Drink a cup of lemon and ginger tea before heading off to sleep – you'll feel much more energized and flatter of tummy by morning.

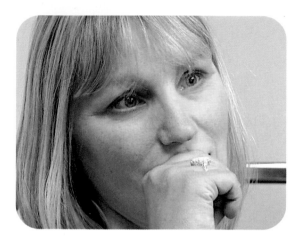

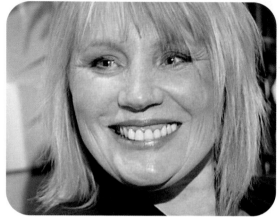

Susan hadn't had her hair cut or styled in a frightening four years – so we sent her off to get some lovely, soft layers worked into her gorgeous blonde hair. With a few lighter shades blended in, she looked years younger. The biggest change was that Susan believed she looked great too. She was looking and feeling much more confident than she had in years and was ready to face the world with her new look. 'I love it!' she said.

A good haircut is always a wise investment: speak to your hairdresser about your needs and lifestyle. There's no point in having a time-consuming haircut that has to be elaborately updated every six weeks if you've got young children, for example. A good hairdresser will help steer you in the right direction and find you a haircut that suits your face shape, as well as your daily schedule.

'I hate my stomach, my hips and my legs. All I see when I look in at my reflection is a fat woman. It's awful. And that's why I've covered myself up.'

HOW TO DRESS BIG BOOBS AND A BOOTILICIOUS BUM

Susan had a classic hourglass shape, which is perfect to dress in 50s style. If you think of Marilyn Monroe and Audrey Hepburn, then you'll have an idea of the style of dressing that best suits this lovely shape. We put her in a bra that fitted correctly and immediately she could see the difference. She had been wearing a 38C bra, when she was actually a 32G. By wearing the correct-size bra she automatically lost six inches from her back, and increased her bust by four cup sizes.

Don't be afraid of being a woman. We got Susan out of her baggy clothes and into softer, girlier fashions to suit her body shape. Well-fitting clothes will hug the hourglass shape's curves. And feminine frocks are the hourglass's best friend, so stop dressing like your fella, and dress to impress him instead.

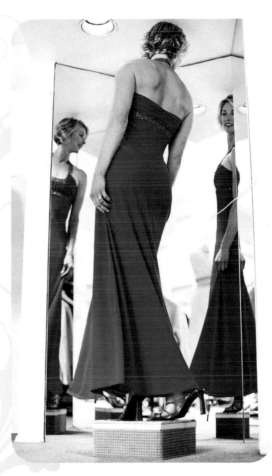

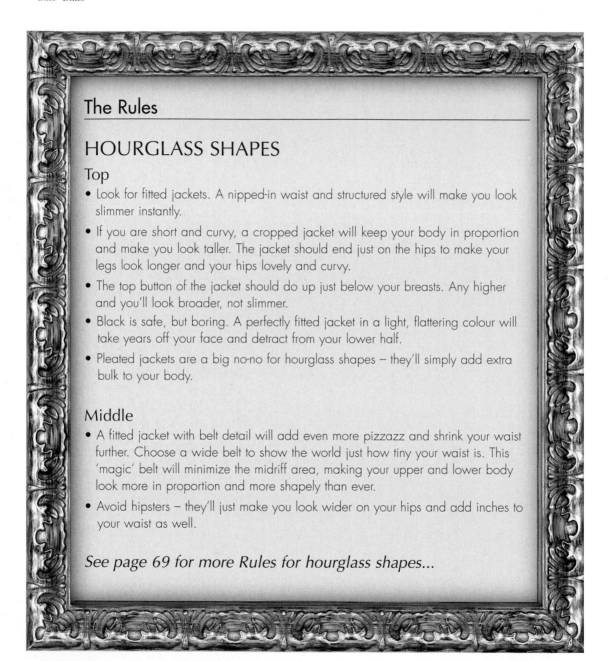

The Rules

HOURGLASS SHAPES

Top

- Look for fitted jackets. A nipped-in waist and structured style will make you look slimmer instantly.
- If you are short and curvy, a cropped jacket will keep your body in proportion and make you look taller. The jacket should end just on the hips to make your legs look longer and your hips lovely and curvy.
- The top button of the jacket should do up just below your breasts. Any higher and you'll look broader, not slimmer.
- Black is safe, but boring. A perfectly fitted jacket in a light, flattering colour will take years off your face and detract from your lower half.
- Pleated jackets are a big no-no for hourglass shapes – they'll simply add extra bulk to your body.

Middle

- A fitted jacket with belt detail will add even more pizzazz and shrink your waist further. Choose a wide belt to show the world just how tiny your waist is. This 'magic' belt will minimize the midriff area, making your upper and lower body look more in proportion and more shapely than ever.
- Avoid hipsters – they'll just make you look wider on your hips and add inches to your waist as well.

See page 69 for more Rules for hourglass shapes...

THE RESULT

When the time came to pose naked Susan really had to draw on all she'd learnt. 'At first I nearly died,' she said. 'But then another part of me inside said "go for it". I felt so good. I just want to skip all around the room. I can't believe that I lay there naked, having my photograph done. And I loved it! I feel so fantastic.'

And Susan's not the only one happy with her look. Her husband Robert is reaping the benefits of his new, sexy and confident wife. Their sex life is back on track and Robert can't believe how beautiful his wife looks. 'You look absolutely gorgeous, absolutely gorgeous,' he said. 'Without a doubt you look very good naked.' Susan's plan post-makeover was to go on holiday with Robert, then come back and fill her wardrobe with nice clothes, dresses, underwear, bags and shoes. Result!

'At first I nearly died. But then another part of me inside said "go for it". I just want to skip all around the room.'

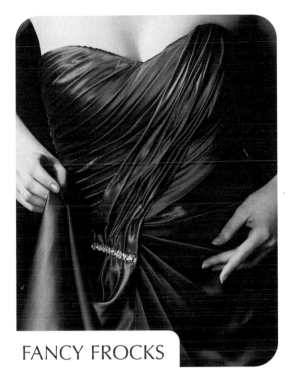

FANCY FROCKS

- Don't be afraid to glam it up. All women, whatever their shape or size, can wear a posh frock – the key is in the cut.
- If you're top-heavy, try a dress that's darker on top to make you look more in proportion on a hot date.
- If you're curvy, a V-neck wrapover dress will flatter your boobs, work your waist and skim those hips – perfect for a sultry summer night.
- If you're slim-waisted with small boobs you'll look great in plunging halter-necks. Dare to wear and you'll always be seen.

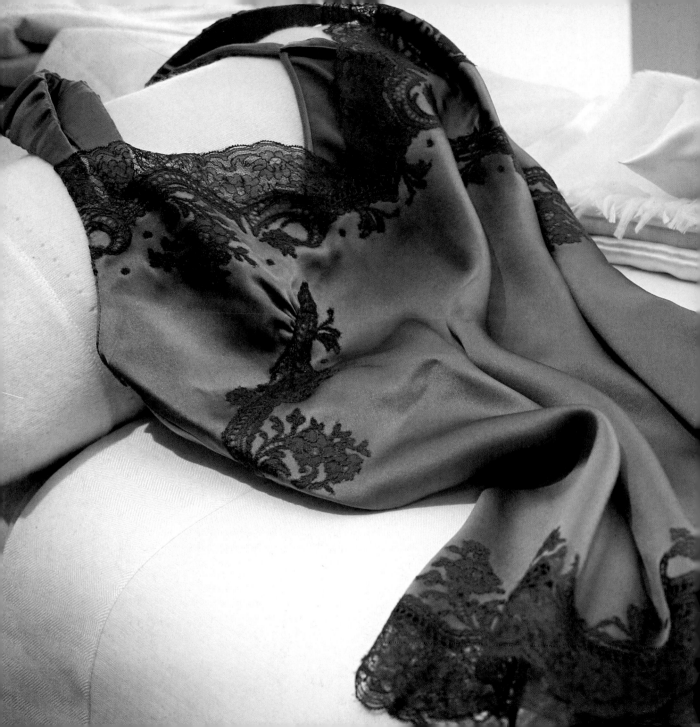

THE THIGH'S THE LIMIT

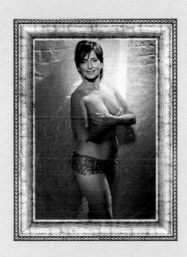

When you're a mother with a busy job, it's easy to put everybody else first. Such was the case with Dorothy Pearlman, 47, a gorgeous woman who had been so busy looking after others that she had almost completely neglected herself. As a result, this nurse and wife hated her appearance: her hair, her thighs and her outfits. Although Dorothy was highly skilled at helping others look and feel better, she was at a loss as to how to apply this kindness to herself.

Dorothy had lost contact with her real self – she had separated her body from her emotions for so long that she was only left with loathing and a feeling of separateness. 'I feel almost asexual – I don't have any va va voom anymore. I used to be a babe and now I'm just a lump.' Her husband Jonathan begged to differ and believed that his wife was one gorgeous mama, who had simply lost confidence. We had to show Dorothy how to treat herself with kindness and respect and discover that under those frumpy clothes there was a yummy mummy just waiting to get out.

WHAT SHE SAW

For Dorothy, taking stock of her appearance was a real struggle. She found it hard to give the attention and focus she had denied herself for so long and felt physically sick looking at her reflection in the mirror. In fact, she had avoided the looking glass for fifteen years!

More than anything else, and like nine out of 10 women, Dorothy loathed her thighs. What's more, she thought that everything she wore made them look worse. When in front of the mirror, she immediately zeroed in on that area of her body. Dorothy's perception of herself was pretty extreme by anyone's standards: 'I've just got to laugh, because if I didn't laugh I would be in tears. I know why I'm here. I'm here because of my thighs. And standing in front of these mirrors only re-enforces why I'm here. They are disgusting, they're fat, they're a funny shape, they're pale. I've got terrible cellulite. They're just horrible. Just vile, vile, vile things.'

Like 70% of women over the age of 40, Dorothy longed for her leaner, toned, younger body and had real difficulty accepting that the figure she had now was due to landmarks in her life: having a child and getting older.

We had a battle on our hands to show Dorothy that looking good naked was about accepting her body and loving all its lumps and bumps, and that dressing her shape was about dressing smart.

BODY PERCEPTION

In our line-up of lovelies, Dorothy had no idea where to place herself. Her thighs – the bane of her life – were in fact a svelte-like 24 inches in diameter. Amazingly, Dorothy judged herself to be the second biggest woman in our line-up, adding an extraordinary ten inches to her thighs in the process. This was a staggering 52% of excess thighage! The truth was that Dorothy was blessed with a gorgeous, womanly figure. The line-up was the first step in getting Dorothy to see that her body was actually sexy and desirable.

'I've got cellulite on my thighs and I just think it's a sad sight.'

THE MAKEOVER

If your thighs, like Dotty, are your least favourite part of your body, then don't despair, as there are clever ways to camouflage them. Straight-legged or wide-legged trousers and jeans give the illusion that your leg is streamlined and toned from hip to heel. Because Dorothy's thighs were slightly wider than her waistline, we advised her to avoid pinstripe or patterned trousers. This is because when a pattern hits a bump it turns into a zigzag and simply highlights the problem area.

Once Dorothy realized that her thigh issue was easily fixed with the right pair of pants, it was time to sort out her top half with correct-fitting underwear. The right type of underwear can help you drop a dress size immediately. Always take the advice of a professional fitter.

Now that we'd smoothed out Dorothy's lumps and bumps without a sniff of the surgeon's scalpel, it was time to show her how to dress her new shape. We chose bright colours and patterns to suit Dorothy's exuberant personality – used cleverly, colour can help accentuate the body parts you love and hide the parts you hate. A particularly successful outfit for Dorothy was a gorgeous smock dress: these are a brilliant way to cover any flabby bits as well as bringing you right up to trend. Matched with a short jacket, all the attention was brought to Dorothy's upper body and away from her dreaded thighs.

Dorothy's verdict was positive too: 'Even though I've got bits that stick out, so what? I'm really, really happy with the way I look.'

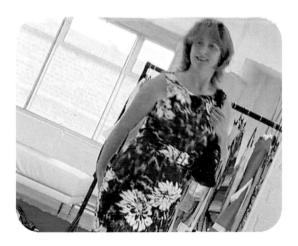
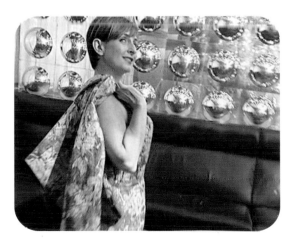

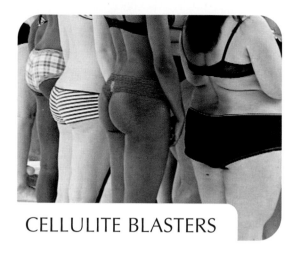

CELLULITE BLASTERS

Cellulite is that lumpy, dimply stuff that appears on your thighs, tummy and upper arms and is caused by fatty deposits under the skin. Even the skinniest of women can get cellulite – it has nothing to do with your weight and all to do with your body and how it distributes fat. The main reasons for cellulite are:

- Not drinking enough water
- Fatty foods
- Smoking
- Drinking coffee
- Overexposure to the sun
- Medication
- Lack of exercise
- Lack of bowel movements
- Stress and hormonal changes

How to banish cellulite

Exercise every day. Just 30 minutes of walking will do wonders for the appearance of your pins. Or you can try skipping, swimming or jogging. It doesn't matter what you do as long as you get that body moving.

While no cream will magic your cellulite away, regular massage and body brushing will help to break up fatty deposits, making your thighs look smoother. Use a natural bristled brush and always brush towards the heart, as this helps to increase your circulation. The better your circulation the less likely you'll suffer from the dreaded orange peel.

Look for products that help the blood flow as well as reduce swelling and improve skin firmness, such as those containing grapeseed extract, pomegranate extract, aloe vera, seaweed and caffeine/green tea (somewhat surprisingly, applying caffeine to the skin does boost circulation). These won't completely banish cellulite, but will help to break up the fatty deposits when massaged firmly in.

Soak in a bath full of detoxifying salts at least once a week for at least 15 minutes. Remember to body brush before getting in the bath. The salts will help to banish excess water and eliminate toxins, which can lead to fatty deposits.

A healthy diet full of richly-coloured vegetables will go a long way to helping your skin look soft and smooth.

Replace your morning coffee with lemon and ginger tea to get your digestive enzymes flowing and help you burn excess waste through the day.

The Rules

PEAR SHAPES

Underwear

- Control pants keep a rein on the thighs while padded briefs transform your bottom from full and flat to pert and peachy.
- Attach special long straps to a strapless bra to pull it down at the back and lift your breasts for fantastic, invisible support.

Top

- Scooped, draped, V-shaped, rounded or square necklines emphasize your bust and draw attention to your face.
- A simple suit dress will flatter. A structured jacket with some glitter will glam it up.
- Wrap tops or a plunging neckline give you much needed oomph up top. Draw the eye away from your bottom with great detailing and accessories.
- A halter-neck top will give the shoulders the width they need, while balancing out the hips and thighs.
- Pear shapes can get away with boob tubes if their shoulders are toned. Go for bright colours to draw the eye upwards.

See page 142 for more Rules for pear shapes...

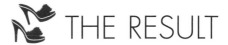

THE RESULT

To finish off Dorothy's new look, we had to do something to tackle those cellulite hang-ups. There's a lot you can do to combat the problem, starting with a good hard look at your diet. See opposite for everything you need to know about the secret of smooth, toned thighs. And remember, even supermodels suffer from cellulite.

With a fake tan application (see p.111) and a body scrub Dorothy felt more pampered than she had in years. Her new outfits brought out the best in her. With clothes, and without them, she finally felt able to face herself and the rest of the world. Despite her misgivings, Dorothy loved her session in front of the photographer, even though she was in her birthday suit!

'It's been an extraordinary experience and I've loved every minute of it. I've felt so special,' she said. 'You don't always want to be centre of attention, but when you are it's amazing. I relaxed into it and I felt really good about myself. Everybody should do this.'

Dresses

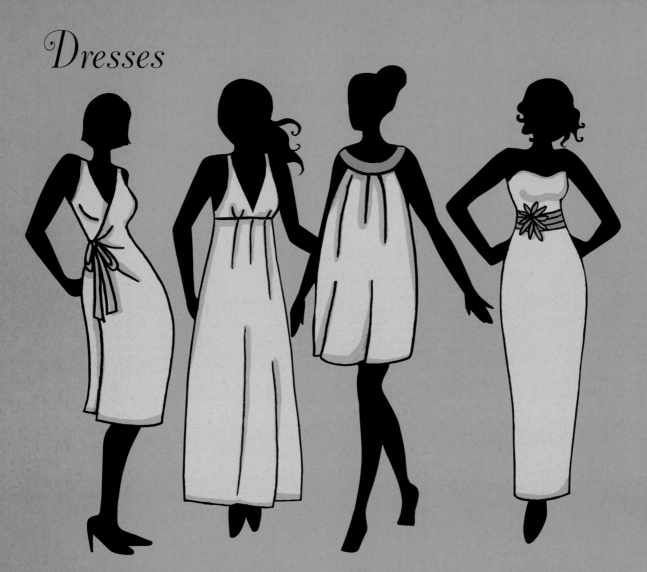

WRAPAROUND

FEATURES: crosses over the chest,
emphasis on the waist
GOOD FOR: all
BAD FOR: none

EMPIRE-LINE

FEATURES: flares from just below
the bust
GOOD FOR: pear, pencil
BAD FOR: hourglass, apple

A-LINE/TRAPEZE

FEATURES: flares from above
the breast
GOOD FOR: apple
BAD FOR: pear, hourglass

STRAPLESS

FEATURES: sits just above boobs
GOOD FOR: hourglass, pencil
BAD FOR: apple

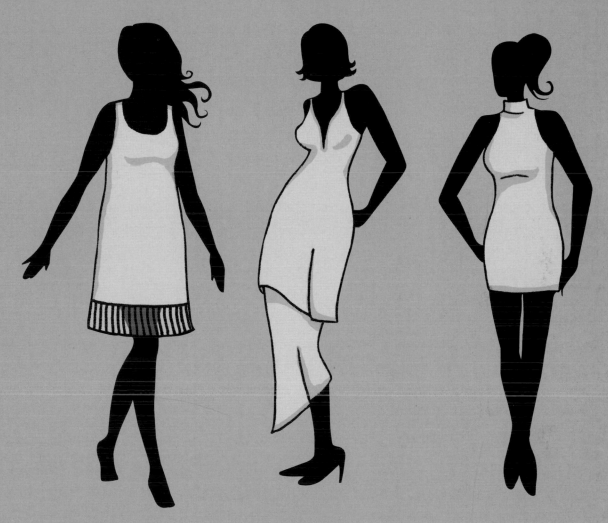

SHIFT
FEATURES: shaped like a rectangle
GOOD FOR: apple, pencil
BAD FOR: pear, hourglass

ASYMMETRICAL
FEATURES: an uneven hem
GOOD FOR: pear, pencil
BAD FOR: hourglass, apple

MINI
FEATURES: short and sweet
GOOD FOR: young, slender shapes
BAD FOR: pear, hourglass

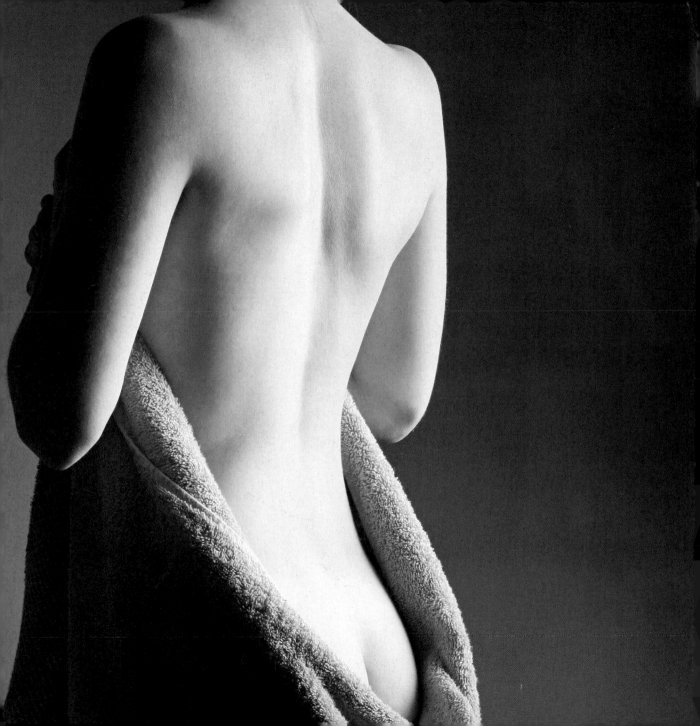

HOW TO LOVE YOURSELF

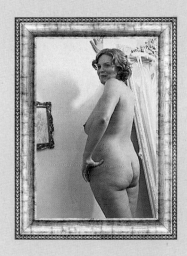

Twins Jeannie and Suzy might have been identical, but they were worlds apart when it came to how they saw themselves. Jeannie Taylor, 29, mother to three children, hated her post-baby body. Even though she and her sister were like two peas in a pod, Jeannie just couldn't see it – she was focusing solely on her flaws and none of her astounding assets.

Jeannie's biggest hang-ups were her breasts and her stretch marks. Her body bore the stresses and strains of childbearing, which Jeannie saw in a negative light. Instead of realizing that her body was a result of her beautiful children, she blamed herself for her body flaws and continually compared herself to her sister. Suzy hadn't had children, so her body shape hadn't changed much over the years.

This constant comparison had taken a toll on Jeannie emotionally. She refused to let anybody in her family see her naked and didn't even like walking down the street with her sister, as she was convinced passers-by were comparing the two of them. We had to show Jeannie that she was just as beautiful as her sister, and that she had a gorgeous look all of her own.

IN THE MIRROR

Jeannie didn't look in the mirror and see herself. Instead, she looked at her identical twin and saw what she believed her body would have looked like had she not had children. 'I used to turn heads. I was proud of it and I loved attracting attention. I've always had big breasts but breastfeeding three children has made them saggy. My stretch marks from my pregnancies have given me a map of lines over my tummy. And I hate them,' she said.

It upset Suzy to see her sister worn down by these pointless comparisons. 'You've had three children,' she said. 'You're still beautiful and that's what I want to hear from you.'

It wasn't just Jeannie's body image that needed a makeover, her wardrobe was crying out for one too. She rarely bought herself new clothes and instead wore Suzy's castoffs. What's more, she still wore her maternity clothing. Whether at the swimming pool, or hitting the

high street, Jeannie followed the rule that more is better. Her swimwear of choice for the pool was a body-covering one-piece with short-style bottoms – which couldn't have been more different from her sister's teeny-weeny string bikini.

We promised Jeannie that after her makeover she would no longer want to be sister, but would be more than happy with what she had.

BODY PERCEPTION

We had to convince Jeannie that her apple-shape body wasn't as large as it seemed in her mind. We showed her and Suzy four cardboard cut-outs of Jeannie's body shape. Only one cut-out was Jeannie's actual shape; the other three cutouts had one to three inches added. Jeannie guessed that Suzy fit in with the second smallest figure, and placed herself at the largest end of

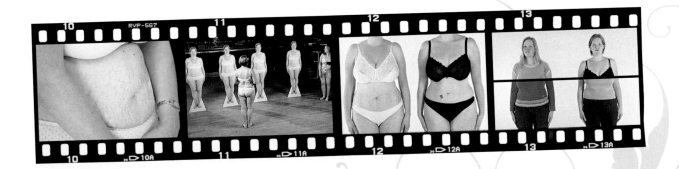

the scale. When she discovered that she was actually smaller than all four cutouts AND smaller than Suzy, she was utterly shocked. And ecstatic! 'I can't believe I'm thinner than Suzy. It's definitely making me feel a bit better!'

We showed strangers a poster of the two sisters and asked them to pick which one had the better body shape.

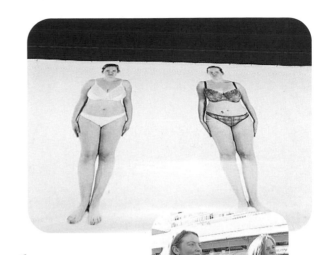

THEY'RE BOTH THE SAME.

I CAN'T TELL THE DIFFERENCE. THEY'RE THE SAME PERSON AREN'T THEY?

YOU WOULDN'T BE ABLE TO PICK WHICH ONE HAD HAD CHILDREN.

DEALING WITH STRETCH MARKS

A whopping 78% of women in this country have stretch marks. That's a sizeable majority. Stretch marks occur when the skin suddenly has to stretch and, as the name suggests, leaves a thin, red mark. This happens most commonly during pregnancy, but can also occur if you suddenly lose or gain weight. Nature does take care of stretch marks and allows them to fade over time, although moisturizing them regularly can help keep the skin supple and smooth.

Body foundation can camouflage body blemishes. But you need to apply it in daylight and using a natural brush. Once you've dabbed on the foundation, cover with powder in your skin shade. This isn't ideal for everyday, but great if you want to cover up your marks when wearing a low-cut dress.

There's nothing you can do to prevent stretch marks during pregnancy, although it's a good idea to rub cocoa butter or almond oil onto your skin. These won't necessarily prevent the marks appearing, but it will help keep your skin soft and supple.

Try to avoid losing or gaining weight too quickly, as this is the second biggest reason why stretch marks appear. If you are on a diet, aim for a weight loss of no more than 2lbs per week. And always, always, always, visit your doctor before beginning a diet to get his or her approval.

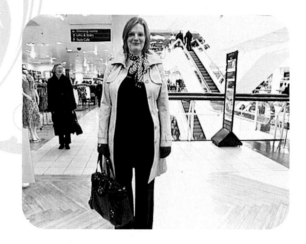

A whopping 90% of you girls aren't confident or comfortable about being naked in front of your friends

THE MAKEOVER

To help Jeannie understand her body shape, we drew an outline of her body shape to show her exactly what it looked like. Jeannie had an apple figure, but with the help of some super dooper structured underpants, we turned her shape into a perfectly proportioned hourglass. The right underwear gave Jeannie a more streamlined figure and helped her lose more than one-and-a-half inches – without having to diet and resort to plastic surgery.

Once we had Jeannie's underwear sorted it was time to dress her for her new body shape, as well as her age and lifestyle. Magic underwear had nipped and tucked Jeannie, so it was time to get back to basics. She'd been

drowning in her sister's hand-me-downs for the past ten years. We needed to find that inner yummy mummy…

We introduced Jeannie to the wonders of tailoring – it's a great way to add a little bit of grown-up dressing to your wardrobe, while emphasizing your fantastic shape. Well-tailored tops that nip in at the waist and fit your chest and back, will take pounds, and years, off you. Team them with wide-legged, flat-fronted trousers and you've got a winning combination. To show Jeannie that her new look didn't need to be too rigid, we teamed her outfit with a pretty trench mackintosh. These wardrobe staples are a great way to emphasize your waist and add a bit of glamour to your everyday look. Jeannie's tailored ensemble had transformed her from frumpy mum to funky mama.

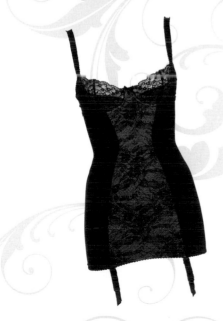

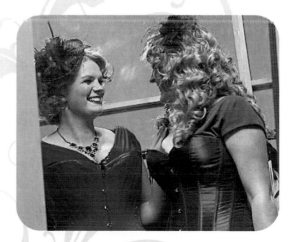

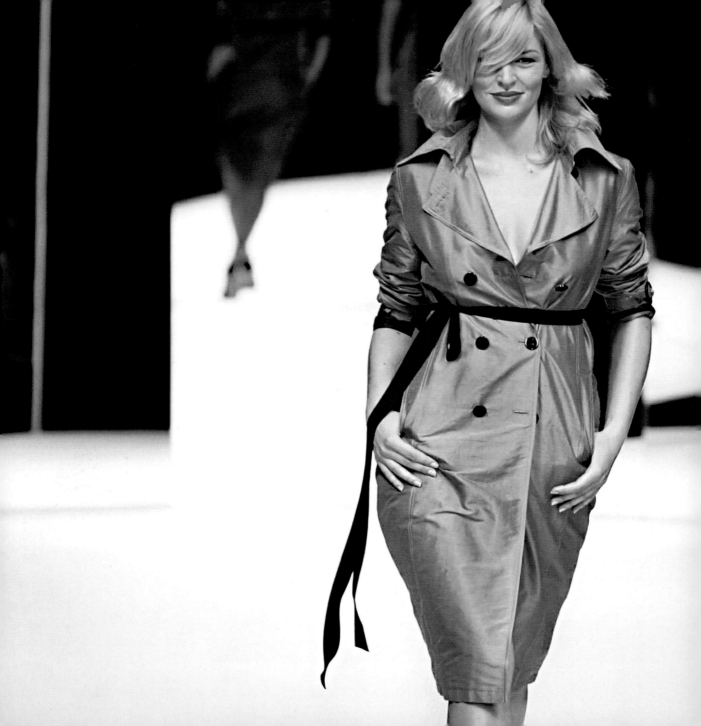

THE RESULT

The tailored clothing really did the trick for Jeannie and gave her such a fantastic shape. She could see it too, despite her initial doubts. She learnt that even 'pull-you-in' tights could be worn every day. 'I've realized that I had to get out of my comfort zone and be brave and it does feel good. I feel sexier, more confident and have learnt to love my body. I've started to turn heads again too!'

Suzy certainly approved: 'You've got such a tiny waist – you look absolutely amazing. Like a film star!'

'I feel sexier, more confident and have learnt to love my body. I've started to turn heads again too!'

Salon Style

SECRET BRIGHTENERS

If you want to camouflage dark circles and highlight those brow bones, then look no further than secret brighteners – or highlighters, as they're generally called. These work by using skin-coloured concealing products to eliminate lines and telltale signs of late nights. To apply skin brighteners properly, it's important to get it right, otherwise you'll just look like you're wearing a mask.

Wear highlighter under your eyes and pay particular attention to your inner eye, just near your nose. Then dab a couple of spots on your brow bone, upper cheekbones and down the centre of your nose. Finish with a dot on your cupid's bow, to make your lips look sexy and full. All makeup should be finished off with a powder – apply lightly with a large, natural-haired brush.

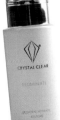

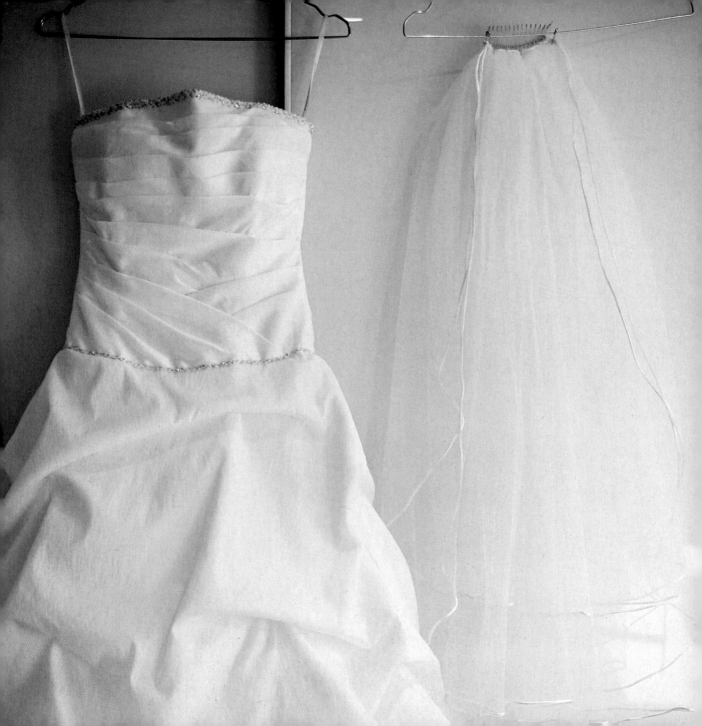

POST-SURGERY BEAUTY

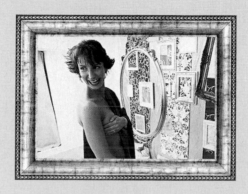

At just 31 years of age, Kelly Chamberlain was diagnosed with breast cancer and subsequently had a mastectomy to remove her left breast. She was fitted with a prosthesis. Breast cancer affects over 46,000 women in Britain each year, a small number of which are aged between 25 and 40. Occasionally the cancer can affect women under the age of 25 too. The effects of breast cancer can be devastating, and the treatment has some very unpleasant side-effects, hair loss being the most common.

Despite fighting cancer, Kelly still felt that the disease had beaten her. Prior to her diagnosis she had been engaged to Toby, but because of her treatment and operation, she had postponed her wedding until she felt that she could be a beautiful bride.

Until Kelly accepted her new body she couldn't get on with her life. Once outgoing and adventurous, post-surgery Kelly hid herself, and her chest, out of view. We had to show Kelly that not only was she a strong, sexy survivor, whose scars were part of her personality and history, but that she could be a babelicious bride and wonderful partner for Toby.

WHAT SHE SAW

When Kelly looked in the mirror, she couldn't see the gorgeous girl staring back at her. All she saw was the scar from her breast cancer surgery, burnt skin from radiotherapy and her once-long hair now short, curly and boyish. Kelly found it very difficult to look at her body in the mirror, as her reflection just reminded her of her cancer ordeal. 'All I see is a body that's let me down,' she said. With her underwear on, Kelly knew that she could disguise her prosthesis, but she was still very aware that she had lost her breast. 'I'm very, very self conscious and cautious about what I wear. But more than that, I look like a different person. I just want to feel pretty again. I don't feel feminine from the neck down and I don't feel feminine from the neck up either.'

> *'I hate the prosthesis, I even hate the word.'*

Whenever Kelly had to wear the prosthesis she was reminded of the cancer. 'Until I can be a beautiful bride for Toby, I'm not interested,' she said. 'I know that Toby says he loves me, for me, but I don't find it sincere, I think it's just a lie. I don't believe that he can find me attractive.' Toby had tried to convince Kelly that the surgery had made no difference to the way he felt about her, but Kelly wouldn't, and couldn't, believe him.

A prosthesis is the most common replacement for a breast, post-surgery and is

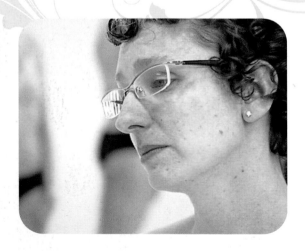

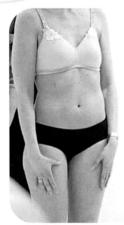

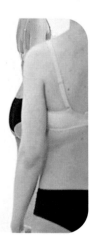

usually worn until reconstructive surgery is done (if done at all). Made out of silicone, it fits into a bra cup and is the same size, skin tone and weight as the natural breast.

We lined up five women who had also had breast cancer. All had undergone surgery and three of them had undergone a full mastectomy. We wanted to show Kelly that not only is it virtually impossible to tell whether somebody fully clothed has had breast surgery or not, but that it is most definitely possible to look sexy and desirable post-surgery. Kelly was unable to tell which women had had surgery, or which were wearing a prosthesis. She was shocked when we revealed the truth to her.

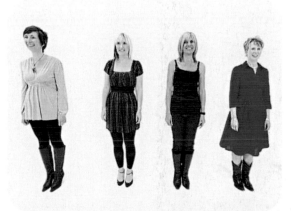

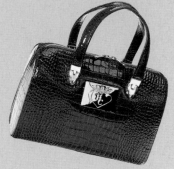

Creating some curves

- If you're self-conscious about your flat chest, then ruffles are the way forward. They flatter all shapes and make your boobs look bigger.
- Soft pastel colours are a clever choice for small-breasted women. And you can team a light-coloured dress with dark tights to emphasize your slim pins.
- Don't forget the details. Floral accessories, bags and quirky heels are what every girl needs – and they'll take attention away from your lack of oomph up top.

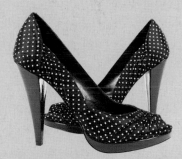

THE MAKEOVER

Kelly wore specially designed bras to hold her prosthesis. While they fulfilled a function, they weren't sexy, and they weren't making Kelly feel like a woman. She described her underwear as 'something your granny would wear'. Kelly had kept all her sexy, more feminine lingerie hidden away in a drawer because she hadn't the heart to get rid of it, even though it was no longer appropriate. She had also hidden her revealing strappy tops, preferring to go out in looser, gathered numbers that hid her breasts.

Kelly's fashion decisions were based around covering up her chest, not coveting the best, and she needed to relearn some basic rules.

We dressed Kelly in a pretty, ruffled dress to help bring back her femininity. The cap sleeves broadened her petite shoulders. The dress also gave her an hourglass shape, which made her

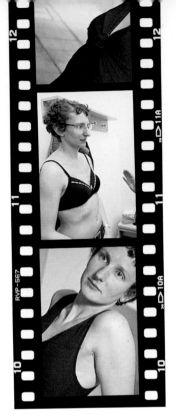

FABRICS FOR YOUR BODY SHAPE

- Velvet – avoid if you're curvy, choose a light velvet instead. Stiffer velvet is good is you're top heavy as it will hold you in and create some support.
- Silk – a lovely way to look more feminine, but wear on the top only, as it creases easily.
- Fringing – a 60s comeback that is great if you're an apple shape as it'll balance out your boobs.
- Ruffles – very tall, thin girls can carry off top-to-toe ruffles, but in the majority of cases, less is more. If you're big breasted, then a ruffle around the waist will balance you out. If you're flat chested, then a ruffled neckline will add some curves.

feel sexy and womanly again. The difference was immediate. Kelly's confidence blossomed and she started to feel like her old self.

We even challenged Kelly to wear a swimsuit – something she'd only dreamt of since her mastectomy. A specially-fitted, plunge-neckline, black swimsuit, with a bespoke pocket sewn in to hold her prosthesis, solved the problem. 'I was so excited when I tried on the swimsuit,' she confessed. 'If someone had shown it to me I would never have tried it on because I'd have said it was too low cut. I didn't think I'd ever feel this good in a swimsuit. I thought the first time I went swimming was going to be hideous, but it's great.'

With the swimwear taboo broken, it was time to challenge Kelly to her greatest test – baring all in a Debenhams store window. The crowd loved it – and loved her body. What's more, the confidence that Kelly gained from her shop window shoot helped her wow the catwalk crowd in her stunning new wedding dress. We'd kept our choice of wedding dress a secret from Kelly until the very last moment. A risk, but luckily she loved it!

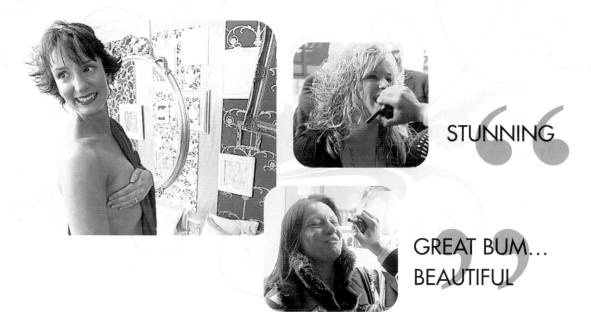

STUNNING

GREAT BUM...
BEAUTIFUL

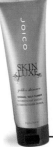

THE RESULT

Kelly had postponed her wedding because she didn't feel she could be a beautiful bride. The wedding dress we found showed off her slim figure, gave her some impact up top and was cut low in the back to reveal a sexy bum. Not only was she ready to walk down the aisle and finally marry Toby, but she also strutted her stuff in a daring, halter-neck red bikini. 'I didn't think I could do it. I wouldn't even open my front door a few weeks ago in my dressing gown. I may have had cancer and a mastectomy, but I can still be a beautiful person. I feel I've conquered the world.'

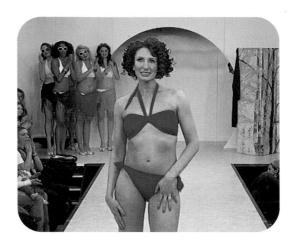

Salon Style

GETTING YOUR BODY READY FOR SUMMER

Use a gradual self-tan. These are moisturizers which contain a self-tanner. Since the pigment isn't as strong as a general self-tanner, you can 'layer' the tan gradually, adding just a little suntan each day. Some even have firming products that will tone those thighs.

Apply some body shimmer. This will help to flash that flesh. You don't have to spend a fortune, the cheap ones do just as good a job. The shimmer will show off the part of your body you want to focus on: collarbone, back, arms, even down the shin bone. But remember girls, less is more.

Finish off with some contouring. Use bronzing powder to add some beautiful shading to your skin tone. Apply on your cheekbones, brow line and collarbones for some seriously sexy shades. Start off with a small amount and add gradually to achieve a perfectly natural look.

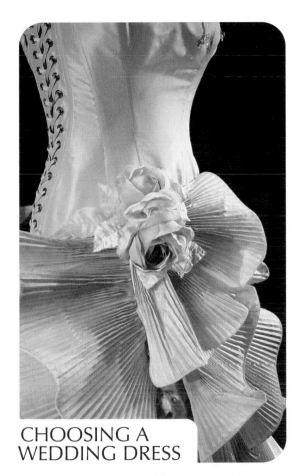

CHOOSING A WEDDING DRESS

Remember that every wedding dress will need to be altered to fit you perfectly. Identify your best asset and find a dress that shows it off. You can still be demure yet daring. Don't be afraid to try new styles.

BIG BOOBS

Busty girls look fab in sweetheart necklines or halter-necks. Boned corsets give fab support and shape. To create a good balance for a heavier bust, go for ball-gown and A-line skirts.

SMALL BUST

Heavily embroidered necklines and busts will flatter your chest and give you sensational curves. A higher neckline is best, as the extra material gives the illusion of beautiful, full breasts.

HOURGLASS SHAPES

Look for detailed necklines for some old-school glamour. Boned corsets will emphasize waspish waists and skirts that skim heavier hips will put the wow into your wedding.

SLIM AND PETITE

Don't go overboard, as ruffles, lace and acres of material will just swamp your little bod. Elegantly cut gowns with empire waists will make your legs look long and slender.

BINGO WINGS

Look for dresses that have a little bolero jacket, or capped sleeves. This will draw attention to your beautiful collarbone and make your arms look long and elegant.

Kelly would like to thank Breast Cancer Care (www.breastcancercare.org.uk), who supported her throughout her journey and during the making of the programme.

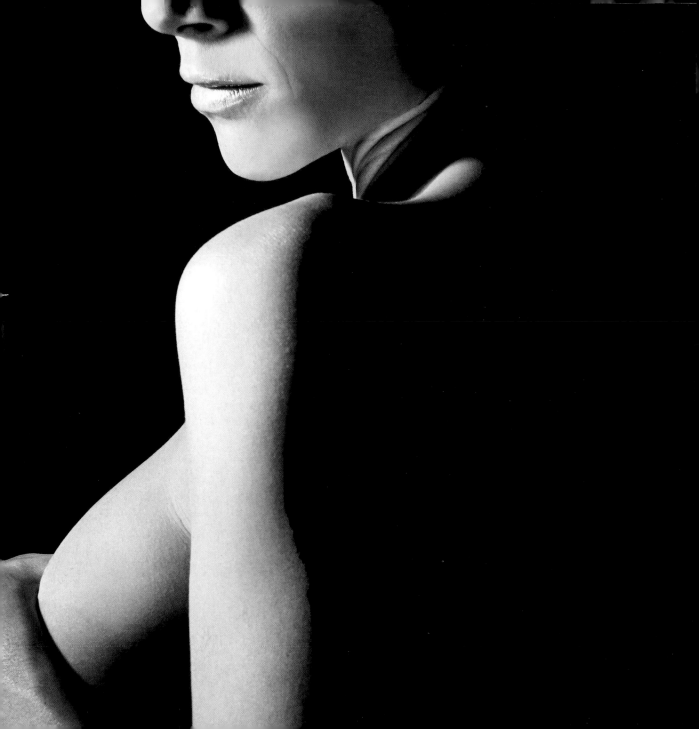

BUST JUST TOO BIG

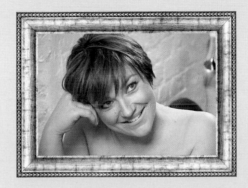

Thirty-seven-year-old Helen Thompson felt like a dowdy housewife. Like many women, she believed that the bodies she saw on television and in magazines were the norm. Perfect figures and perfect boobs. Deep down she knew it was all fake, and yet this is what she measured herself against. Helen hated her breasts most of all and thought they were too big and busty, even though her husband Gary disagreed. 'Since having children my body has gone horribly wrong. I now see an ugly fat person,' she said. 'When they hand you your babies, it's as if they take away a bit of that confidence that you had.' She thought that her body was so fat, and that she was so ugly, that she refused to let even her children see her naked. She was contemplating surgery to reduce the size of her breasts.

Helen's negative body image was affecting all aspects of her life. Her self-esteem was even damaging her career and influencing the type of job she could apply for. Once a high-flying career woman, she now lacked the confidence to return to her former working-girl glory. We set out to help convince Helen that her boobs were actually one of her greatest assets. Once we got that sorted, her confidence soared and the worn-out housewife was ready to be transformed into a catwalk diva.

IN THE MIRROR

Before appearing on the show, Helen avoided full-length mirrors at all costs. 'I feel very exposed when I see myself in the mirror. I just hate my enormous bosoms so much, I don't want to look at them,' she said. Her boobs were the bane of her life. 'I just feel incredibly old and incredibly wide. I want to see somebody who feels good about herself. Who can take her clothes off and say, hey, this is me.'

Helen believed that surgery was the only way to improve her post-baby body. The truth is that although around 15,000 women have surgery each year to reduce the size of their bust, many could avoid the expensive and painful operation just by investing in bras that fit correctly. She also hated her broad shoulders, which made her feel unfeminine. Her confidence was at an all-time low. 'It's wrapped up in how I see myself and has grown into a bit of self-loathing,' she admitted.

'I've never liked my boobs, and there's no way I ever will like them.'

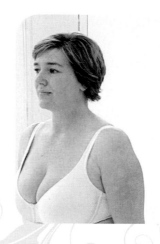 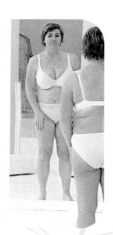

BODY PERCEPTION

British women have the largest breasts in Europe – the average bra size is now a generous 36C. Helen's breasts are two sizes larger than the national average, at 36E, but even so, she's still not as big as she thinks she is. In a line-up of women with breast sizes ranging from E to J, Helen positioned herself four sizes larger than she actually is, which gives an idea of how distorted a view of herself she had.

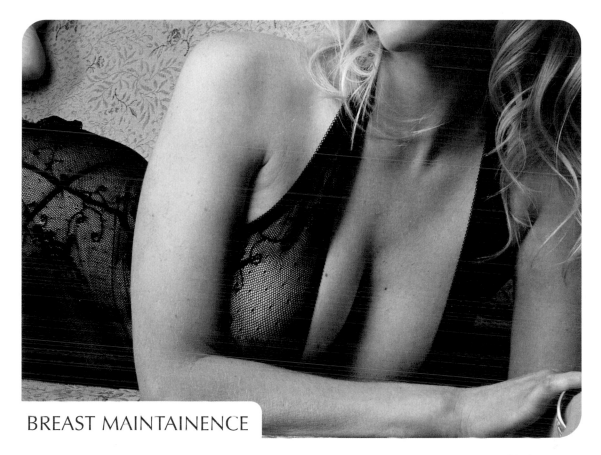

BREAST MAINTAINENCE

- A bust-firming gel won't make much difference to your boobs, so just use your usual body moisturizer and use the money you save towards investing in some well-fitting underwear.

- The breasts are made of fat and tissue, not muscle. So as you get older, your breasts get droopier. But wearing a good bra, and a sports bra when you exercise, will help stop your boobs going south.

- Bust-firming treatments work by sending electric shocks to pull the muscles up. It's not for wimps but it works.

- Body wraps can also achieve similar results as surgery – they're a great treatment to try before baring all.

Balancing your boobs with your bum

Top

- If you're top heavy, balance out your shape with soft materials and cuts, such as a cowl-neck top.
- Shirts and tops with a built-in waistband create the illusion of curves and make you look taller as the waistband separates your upper body from your legs, giving you a longer-looking torso.
- Wraparound blouses and shirts are your new best friends. Tie them tight to show off your waist.
- Jersey or stretch material is great for well-endowed girls, as you can adjust it easily to fit your boobs.
- Darker colours are ideal if you want to seem slimmer.
- Long, dangly earrings will elongate your neck and transform you from duckling into swan.

Middle

- Always wear outfits that taper at your waist to stop you looking shapeless. There's no point in having a killer body if you hide it under shapeless clothes.
- A softly tailored jacket that nips in at the waist is a wardrobe must.

Bottom

- Balance killer cleavages with A-line skirts to create a sexy, hourglass shape.
- Tailored trousers that fit correctly are a wise investment.
- A bold print below the waist will balance out slim-hipped, big-breasted women who want to add curves.
- High heels will give you va-va-voom and further balance your silhouette.

THE MAKEOVER

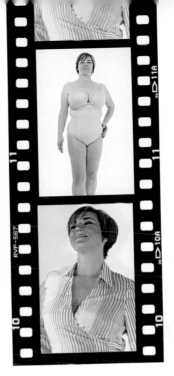

Helen's hourglass body puts her in the same category as many of the Hollywood glamour pusses who had the world drooling over them in the 50s and 60s. We made the most of her screen siren shape by dressing her in a full-length halter-neck dress, which helped her embrace her natural curves. The halter top will always help you project a 'who-gives-a-damn' attitude, whether you're pear-shaped, hourglass or a big-bottomed beauty. If you're wearing an unusual neckline such as a halter-neck then choose a multiway bra, which can be transformed into a halter bra just by removing one strap. This sexy support lifted Helen's breasts and gave her a stunning silhouette. The dress then nipped in tightly at her waist, before skimming her hips. Teemed with some teetering heels, Helen was ready to wow the crowds.

KNICKER KNOW-HOW: SEXY OR MAGIC?

Every woman should have two types of underwear: sexy and magic. The sexy stuff is for obvious reasons – it makes you and your lover feel fantastic. But magic knickers are all about helping clothes fall better on your body, no matter what your size or your shape. Forget plastic surgery – magic pants are the only money you need to spend. Some just control your tummy and butt, others squeeze you in right up to your bra, and down over your thighs (see p.171 for more). No-one's going to pretend that magic knickers are much of a turn-on, but that's why you have the sexy pants too!

As for your top half, minimizer bras can be a good option if your boobs are out of control. They flatten your boobs out and can make you look two sizes smaller. If, on the other hand, you're brave enough to draw attention to your breasts, opt for a plunge bra. It'll give you a classic cleavage and hoist those babies up.

THE RESULT

With her super-sexy dress, fab heels and siren-style hair and make-up, Helen could strut her stuff on the catwalk in front of thousands of people – even her mother! All she had to do was hold her head high, pull her shoulders back and tummy in, and she was model-ready. 'Modelling in my lingerie was scarier than the nude shoot, but I felt gorgeous and lovely,' she said. 'It's incredible. It doesn't feel like me. This isn't how I dress. I didn't think I could look like this at all.'

65% of UK women would rather be curvy than skinny.

Salon Style

EXFOLIATING

If you're going to be butt-naked, it's essential that your skin looks as gorgeous and glowing as it possibly can. An all-over body exfoliator is a must, but if you can afford a professional body scrub down, it'll be well worth it.

If you don't want to spend money on an exfoliator then rummage around your kitchen cupboards instead. Add a handful of salt to some olive oil and rub it all over for silky soft skin.

Body brushing is also an essential beauty routine. Using a loofah, or long-handled body brush, actually 'brush' your skin towards your heart in long, sweeping movements. This boosts the circulation and smoothes out any surface blemishes.

After you've exfoliated all over, apply a fake-tan. You'll immediately look as if you've stepped off the beach and will even make those thighs and waist look slimmer.

Don't forget to apply moisturizer to towel-dried skin to help keep your body butt and smooth.

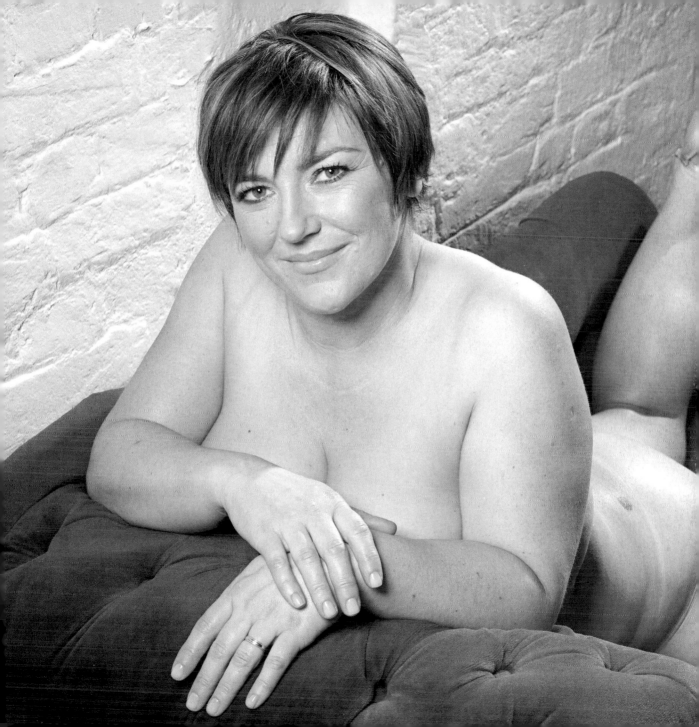

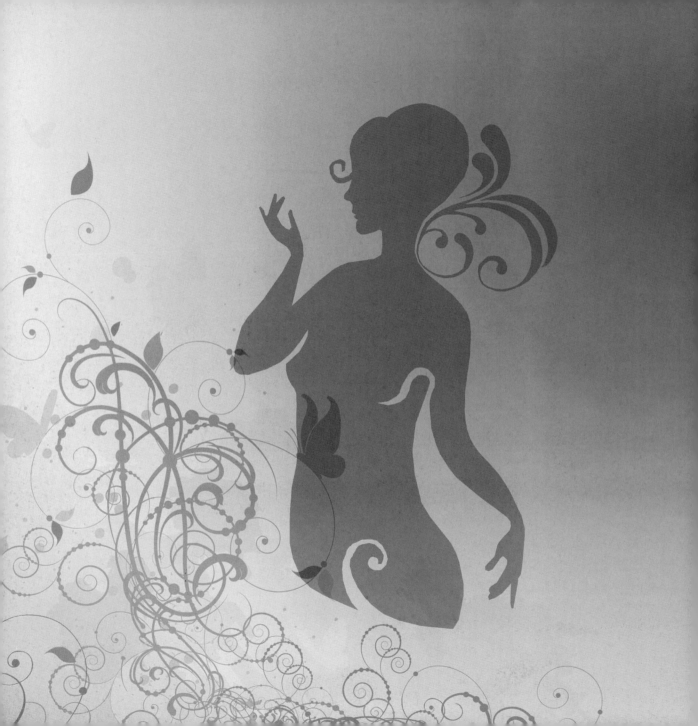

Chapter 3

TUMMY TROUBLES

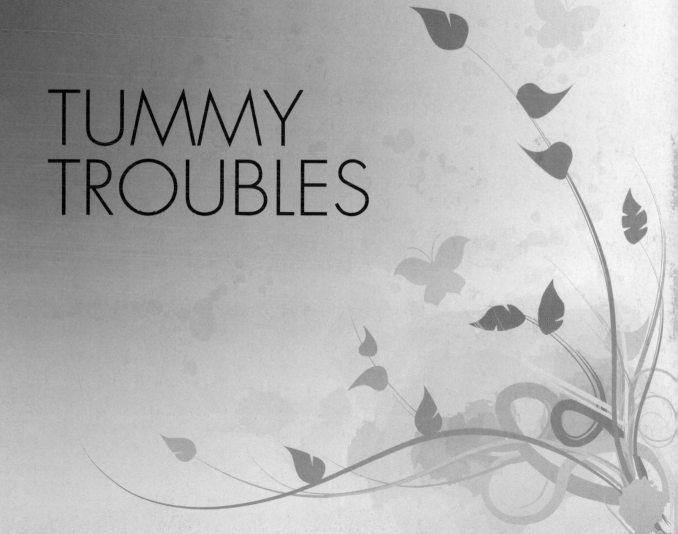

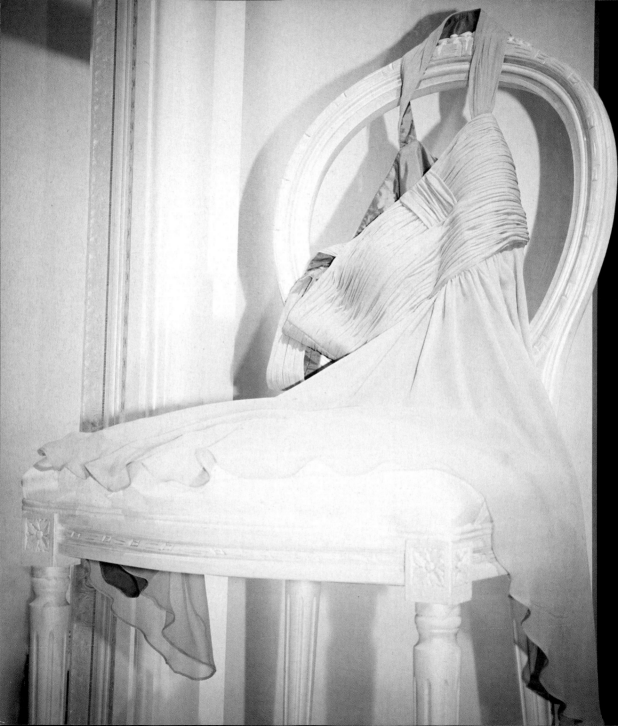

TAMING THE TUMMY

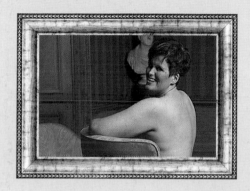

The hourglass figure is the most inspirational and envied body shape of all. That should come as no surprise. It is exquisitely feminine. Yet hourglass girls consistently fail to both recognize their wonderful shape or wear the clothes that will do justice to those curves.

Forty-four-year-old Debbie Onions came on the show with a very poor body image, which had badly affected her self-esteem. Yet what Debbie had achieved was already pretty amazing – she had gone from a size 26 to a size 16, and was working as a slimming instructor, helping to motivate others to lose weight. Despite this, she still thought she was overweight, unattractive and felt a fraud. Behind her confident front, Debbie still saw herself as a fat girl.

Our mission was to show her just how fabulous she was and how to make the most of her womanly curves. We wanted this sexy singleton to stop spending her nights on the sofa and start strutting her stuff out in the big wide world.

IN THE MIRROR

When Debbie looked in the mirror all she saw was her flabby stomach and hips. 'It's horrible,' she said, 'like I'm wearing a big apron'.

And yet Debbie the career woman was a confident, outgoing person, inspiring others to to lose weight as she had managed to do so successfully herself. 'I think I come across as very confident in my job,' she said, 'but privately I'm the complete opposite. I want to take that confident feeling I project in my work and apply it to my personal life. If I could do that, there'd be no stopping me.'

Debbie felt that, despite all her hard work, she simply didn't look the way women are supposed to look. Like many of us, she'd spent far too much time looking at images of women in magazines and wondering why she looked different from them.

'You're supposed to be all nice and flat. You're supposed to be slim and slender, nice and pretty. Not big like this,' she said.

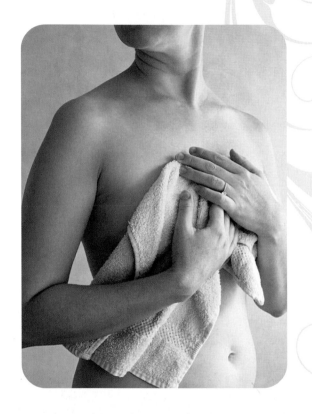

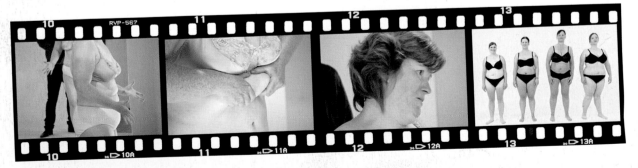

BODY PERCEPTION

Debbie hated the area just under her breasts – her top tummy. She was actually a very average 37 inches, but in the line-up she placed herself as the biggest girl. In fact, Debbie had the second smallest midriff in the line-up. She'd been adding inches onto her body in her head and had no idea of how slim and sexy she really was.

Debbie's dislike of her body wasn't about her weight, but about liking the person inside. Our job was to show Debbie how to dress to make the most of her body, so that when she looked in that mirror, she'd love what she saw.

87% of women say they're unhappy with their weight. No matter what that weight is!

Glamour bras

Underwear is the most important part of your outfit. The wrong underwear can make even the most stylish of outfits look wrong for your shape.

There's no reason that girls who are heavy up top shouldn't wear glamorous and sexy bras and there are plenty of companies out there that cater specifically for you.

- The plunge bra is the best non-surgical way to lift your boobs and create a sexy cleavage.
- If you're wearing a backless dress, then opt for a bare-all, backless bra.
- For maximum flexibility in your bras, choose a multiway. These can be worn in various ways to suit your outfit.

Whatever you do, ladies, make sure you get the right size for your breasts. Visit a underwear store and get yourself measured. You'll be surprised by what size you really are.

THE MAKEOVER

Debbie had no chance of ever getting noticed while she still dressed as someone who was 20 stone plus. She had a gorgeous little body, and had worked hard to lose that weight. Once Debbie could get rid of the 'fat girl' in her head, she'd start to look and act more confident.

The secret was to dress her hourglass shape properly. That would enable Debbie to see how stylish she could really be, then she would start to *believe* herself to be that slim, sexy, confident woman. Dressing her shape would allow the pounds to drop off her.

No matter what your shape there's a style and outfit out there that will make you look, and feel, fantastic.

HOURGLASS FIGURE KNOW-HOW

The hourglass shape is pretty easy to dress once you understand the rules. A typical hourglass figure has:

- similar width hips and shoulders;
- a tiny waist;
- long and elegant arms;
- shapely calves and ankles.

If you're carrying a bit of extra weight around your bust, upper midriff and thighs, then accentuate your thinnest part. This is your

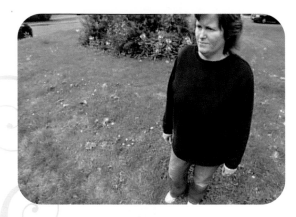

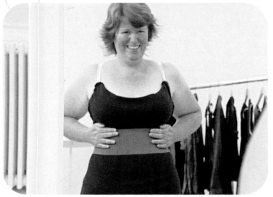

collarbone, where you probably don't have any excess flesh. Flash this flesh to the world and nobody will be looking at your thighs – they'll be staring at your daring décolletage.

Debbie had been hiding a fabulous figure. By uncovering those curves and showing off that tiny little waist we boosted her confidence and managed to show her what she *really* looked like.

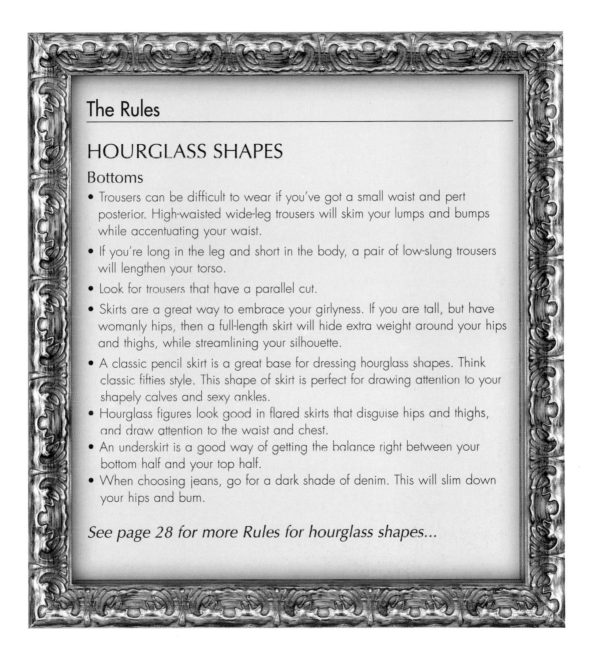

The Rules

HOURGLASS SHAPES

Bottoms

- Trousers can be difficult to wear if you've got a small waist and pert posterior. High-waisted wide-leg trousers will skim your lumps and bumps while accentuating your waist.
- If you're long in the leg and short in the body, a pair of low-slung trousers will lengthen your torso.
- Look for trousers that have a parallel cut.
- Skirts are a great way to embrace your girlyness. If you are tall, but have womanly hips, then a full-length skirt will hide extra weight around your hips and thighs, while streamlining your silhouette.
- A classic pencil skirt is a great base for dressing hourglass shapes. Think classic fifties style. This shape of skirt is perfect for drawing attention to your shapely calves and sexy ankles.
- Hourglass figures look good in flared skirts that disguise hips and thighs, and draw attention to the waist and chest.
- An underskirt is a good way of getting the balance right between your bottom half and your top half.
- When choosing jeans, go for a dark shade of denim. This will slim down your hips and bum.

See page 28 for more Rules for hourglass shapes...

THE RESULT

To complete Debbie's look, we cut her hair to flatter her jawline – immediately she lost pounds and her beautiful eyes were highlighted. Then a full-body massage, manicure, pedicure and Debbie was ready to go.

From frumpy to fabulous. Debbie was transformed from a woman ashamed of her 'old' self to a girl-about-town who couldn't wait to kick up her heels.

Debbie learnt to love her curves, and how to dress to show them off to their best advantage. Now when she looks in the mirror she sees exactly what's reflected: a beautiful woman with curves to match.

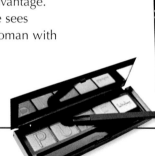

Salon Style

COLOUR IT RIGHT

If you have auburn hair like Debbie then make the most of your Jessica Rabbit features:

Make freckles part of your look.

Use neutral eyeshadow so you don't overpower your features with colour. Brown and peach shadow are best.

Brown-based red lipsticks flatter redheads better than peach or pinky-reds.

Don't forget your eyeliner and mascara. Redheads tend to have pale lashes, so use these little beauties to draw attention to your pretty peepers.

LAYERING FOR HOURGLASS GIRLS

The layered look worked particularly well for Debbie's body shape, but it can be difficult to get right. Here are some tips:

- Keep to thin fabrics and add bulk with scarves and belts.
- Don't be afraid to mix your textures – these keep your look interesting.
- Wear a corset. This will cinch in your tiny waist even further.
- Wear an underskirt to bulk out your waist in a feminine way and balance our your boobs.
- A black and white evening dress screams 'glamour'. Add matching accessories to pull the whole look together.

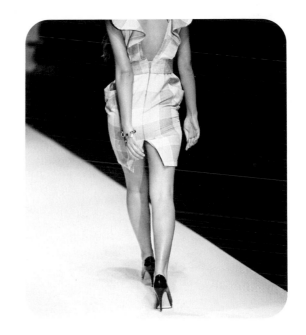

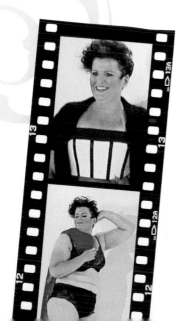

'My confidence is sky high. If you can walk with your shoulders pulled back, your chin up, a good pair of heels and a bit of lippy — that's all you need!'

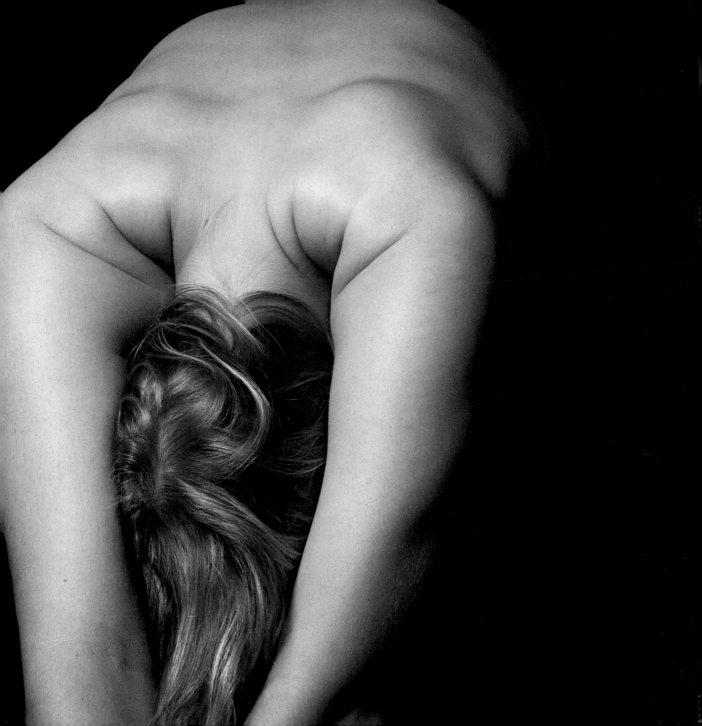

POST-BABY GLOOM

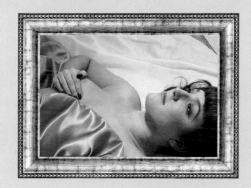

Mum-of-one Vikki Brace, 28, has taken the term 'stay at home mum' to the extreme. Since having her baby she had hidden herself away and even at the height of summer preferred to slob out in jeans and jumper rather than flaunt her flesh in some flirty skirts.

When Vikki had her baby, which was more than two years before we met her, she left her body confidence in the delivery room. She was so caught up with her negative body image that she refused to get naked – even in front of her adoring husband Mark. She locked herself away in the bathroom if he was in the bedroom, and it had been a shocking four years since he had last seen her naked. Vikki kept photographs of herself in a bikini from her pre-baby days stuck to the refrigerator, so that she felt bad about herself all the time. Her lack of confidence wasn't helped by having a twin sister, whose presence reminded Vikki of what she would look like if she hadn't had a baby. We needed to convince her that the extra pounds added since her baby's birth should be celebrated not hated.

WHAT SHE SAW

When Vikki was confronted with her naked self it was an emotional and harrowing experience for her. She described her body as like dough – lumpy, bumpy and with love handles. Yet she actually had a great hourglass figure hiding under all those frumpy outfits. Almost every new mum feels pressure to be back in their skinny jeans just days after having their baby – and we see so many pictures of celebrities doing just that. Yet having a baby is not the end either for your body or your wardrobe. Quite the opposite, it should be the making of you as a woman.

Vikki's husband Mark couldn't even remember the last time he'd seen his wife naked. 'Vikki has her own idea of what she looks like and it's impossible to convince her otherwise,' he said. 'If Vikki got her confidence back, she'd get back to the person she was.'

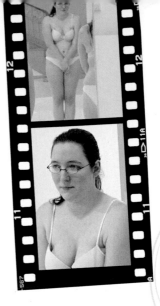

Feeling at ease with your naked body is the first step to getting back on the road to body acceptance. We had to get Vikki back and show how to look and feel blooming marvellous.

Like 8 out of 10 new mums, Vikki's biggest body hatred was her muffin top. She thought her overhang was so huge, it had really taken over

THE BEST SKIRTS FOR YOUR LEGS

- Big thighs – knee-length skirts will skim over the tops of your legs and show off the more slender parts of your legs.
- Thin pins – mini skirts are perfect for long, lean and toned legs.
- Petite – mid-length skirts will maximize your leg length without making you look out of proportion
- Pear shape – A-line skirts that skim your hips are perfect.
- Straight up and down – tulip skirts will add volume to your hips.
- Hourglass – knee-length pencil skirts will give you a 'sexy secretary' shape.

her life. When we asked Vikki to judge her own measurements, she gave herself an extra 4 inches. The discovery that she was actually much slimmer than she thought had a dramatic effect on Vikki, but it was only the first step.

THE POSTER TEST

Vikki's body confidence needed a big boost and what better way than to ask the British public what they thought of her? She needed to realize that other people didn't think that she was fat and unattractive.

"SHE'S GOT A LOVELY HOURGLASS FIGURE.

NOT FAT MUMMY – YUMMY MUMMY. SHE'S GOT A LOVELY TUMMY."

"I THINK SHE'S BEAUTIFUL.

THE MAKEOVER

Around 25% of new mums say they want cosmetic surgery. But there's no need to go under the knife to get a new body – mums can still have killer style.

If you're conscious of your post-baby tummy, tailored clothes are made for you – and they're much cheaper and quicker than plastic surgery when it comes to creating flat tummies and beautiful boobs.

We had to get Vikki out of her tracksuit bottoms and into sexy skirts to show off her hourglass figure. We chose A-line skirts with vertical patterns and wide waistbands. These made her look taller, slimmer and shapelier, and helped hold in her tummy. On her top half we chose wraparound blouses and cardigans, which accentuated her tiny waist gave her a sexy edge. A tailored jacket gave her an even more eye-catching waistline. Perfect for running errands and meeting other mums for coffee.

After some pampering, body maintenance and a brand new haircut that brought her hair to her shoulders and gave her a fringe to show off her beautiful eyes, Vikki was good to go.

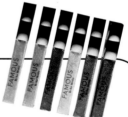

Salon Style

LUSCIOUS LIPS

It's essential to keep your lips looking gorgeous – you'll never know when you might be using them…

If you're going for a natural look, then match your lipstick to the colour inside your lips. Pull your bottom lip out and check out that colour!

If you want something more dramatic, such as red, then the rest of your make-up should be toned down.

Apply a concealer to the entire lip area to create a base. Then, outline your lips in a neutral lip colour. Apply the lipstick and then blot with a tissue and add one more layer. To get rid of any excess, put a finger in your mouth and pull it out.

Add highlighter in your pout to make your lips look bigger and plumper.

THE RESULT

It was interesting that, as it gradually dawned on Vikki that she could look good – with or without clothes – she began to enjoy her mothering role more. She started taking baths with her baby girl Emily, and to feel more natural about exposing her body. But how did she feel about the new her? 'I feel a million dollars. I really do. I feel sexy, glamorous and feminine. I'm really happy. Even on my wedding day I didn't look like this.' Husband Mark was impressed too: 'I'm seeing more than I've seen before,' he said. 'She's no longer running into the bathroom to get changed, but is showing her body off in the bedroom.'

Vikki had finally clicked that it's okay to love yourself. She didn't care what anybody else thought (for the record, they thought she looked great) and was confident that she looked good – any time, any place.

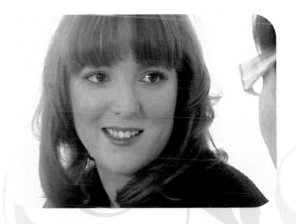

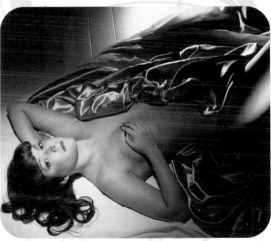

'I feel sexy, glamorous and feminine. Even on my wedding day I didn't look like this.'

YOUR ALL-DAY PAMPER

Vikki had a body firming treatment that not only pampered her post-baby skin, but also gave her some much-needed time for herself. If you want to have some pampering without the salon prices, try our mini spa day below. It will have you feeling on top of the world.

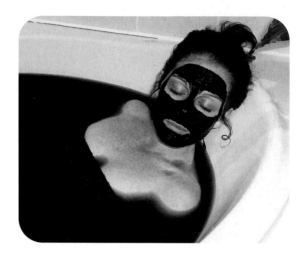

7am Wake up and drink a glass of warm water with lemon juice to get your circulation going.

8am A healthy porridge or muesli for breakfast will fill you up till lunchtime.

9am Using a body brush, brush your naked body from toe to shoulder, always aiming towards the heart.

10am Jump in the shower and exfoliate your body all over. You should feel the tingles from head to toe.

11am Get outdoors. A brisk walk to the park or even to buy your favourite magazine will get some roses into your cheeks and firm that bottom.

12pm Time for some pampering. Give yourself a manicure and pedicure (see p.100). Your feet and hands should be beach-ready at all times.

1pm Lunchtime. Enjoy a bowl of soup and wholemeal roll.

2pm Naptime. It's your day off, so go and visit the land of nod

3pm Time to get up! And get moving! Pop on some music and dance around, or if you have a fitness DVD follow this for around 30 minutes.

4pm Rest time. Fill the bath with warm water and add one tablespoon of Epsom salts. Turn the phone off, light some candles and soak your worries away. Add a face and hair mask for some extra pampering treats.

5pm Fake it! Fake tan will help you look thinner, more toned and healthier. Then apply moisturizer to your whole body.

6pm A healthy wholesome dinner is a must. Try chicken with rice and vegetables for a filling nighttime meal. A pudding of fruit and yoghurt will give you that sweet hit you're craving.

7pm Pop your favourite movie on the DVD and curl up for some good old-fashioned 'me' time.

10pm It's an early night for you! You'll wake up feeling fresh-faced, refreshed and fabulous.

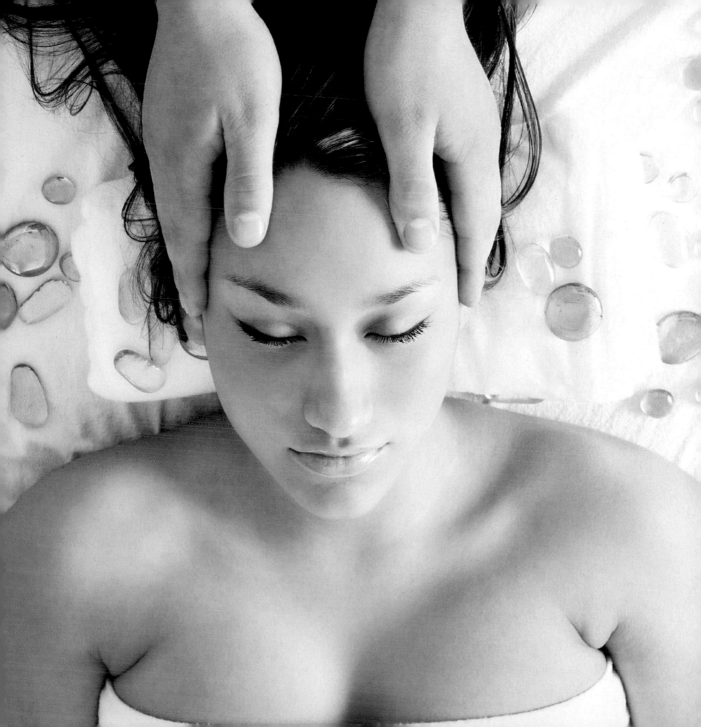

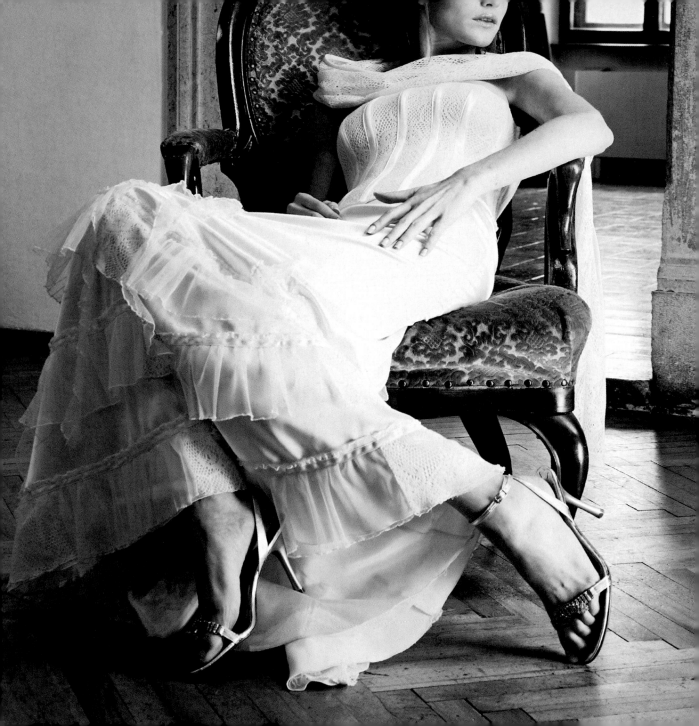

TUMMY TURMOIL

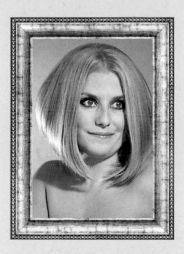

Liz Marlowe, 29, lived with her husband Adrian and her two young children in High Wycombe, Berkshire. As a size 16, Liz was perfectly in line with the national average. Yet she was so down on herself that she wouldn't even strip off in front of her hubby.

Liz used to be a blonde bombshell who made an impact wherever she went. But she had turned from a bright and beautiful English rose into a wilting wallflower. Her wardrobe could be summed up in three words: fleeces, t-shirts and jeans. Liz's husband thought that she was gorgeous and beautiful, but there was no convincing her of that fact. Her hatred of her body shape had become so bad that she had begun to worry that it would affect her young daughter's self-image too. Liz also believed that her husband secretly thought she should lose weight, despite his constant reassurances to the contrary.

We needed to boost Liz's confidence and make her realize that she wasn't the misshapen blob she thought she was. First step was to get Liz out of her usual clothes and get her actively living a more fashionable, fabulous life.

IN THE MIRROR

Liz found it extremely difficult to look at her reflection in the mirror. When we forced her to confront the glass she couldn't see any part of her body that she liked and just wanted to go home! 'I want to change everything from the top of my head to the tips of my toes,' she said. 'Everybody else I see looks thinner, prettier, and more stylish than me.' The last time Liz had seen herself in a full-length mirror was about eighteen months earlier. She just couldn't face it. 'It's about confronting your demons. It's far easier to hide your body than it is to take a good look and accept it.'

Liz's biggest fear was that her daughter would grow up with the same body loathing as she suffered, and that she'd also be ashamed of her body. Liz wanted to be confident enough to uncover her body, and teach her daughter how to love herself, no matter what.

Adrian was desperate to get the old Liz back: 'She is the mother of my two wonderful

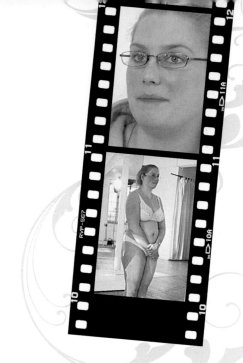

children. I cannot hold her low self-esteem against her. I want to help her in any way I can,' he said.

BODY PERCEPTION

The first step to body confidence is to get your body shape and size into perspective. In a row of six women, Liz judged her waist to be five inches larger than it really was. That's two dress sizes. Her waist measurement was actually 40 inches, which was smaller than all the other girls present. Liz was shocked to discover that she was the smallest woman in the line-up, but delighted to find out what her body measurements really were.

60% of women prefer lights off when they get naked.

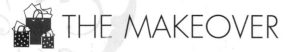

THE MAKEOVER

Liz had a combined pear/hourglass body shape. This means having slightly smaller shoulders than waist and hips. Like many women who don't like their bodies, Liz made the common mistake of wearing clothes that were far too big for her. This just made her look out of proportion and gave no hint of the goddess hiding under those fleeces. We ended up dressing her in clothes that were three sizes smaller than the stuff in her wardrobe. The key to balancing out her hips was to emphasise her knockers. This in turn meant her waist looked smaller and slimmer.

With the correct underwear for her shape – those magic knickers again – we had the foundations sorted. The magic underwear gave Liz back some control. 'I have a waist and a fairly flat tummy now,' Liz exclaimed.

Liz had a tendency to put weight on her bum and thighs, so we shopped carefully for trousers and found a pair that skimmed her thighs. We dressed her in a pair that had a clever built-in support waist and a crease down the front of the leg. Voila! She looked three sizes smaller.

Fishnets proved a great way to add some femininity to her outfit and made her legs look thinner and sexy. A wrap dress in a pretty summer print brought a smile to Liz's face and put a spring in her step.

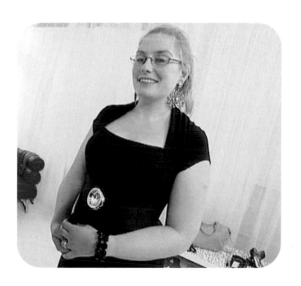

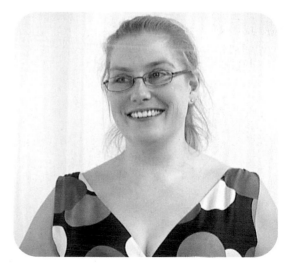

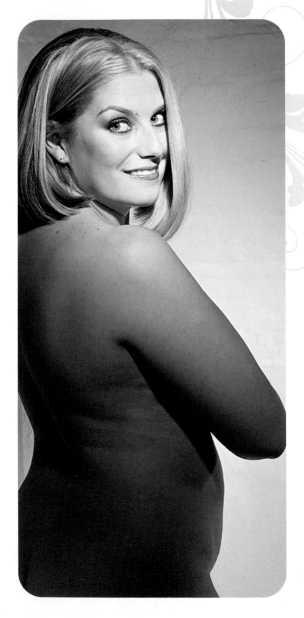

The final touch? We cut Liz's long locks into a face-framing bob that screamed sophistication as well as fabulous fun. Some lighter highlights and darker lowlights gave depth and movement to her beautiful barnet. Liz's eyes were her flirtiest feature so we added some smokey shadow to enhance them. It's always a good idea to accentuate one facial feature, whether it's your eyes, lips or cheekbones. And remember, you tell people more about how happy you are in your body just by your walk – you really don't need to say a word.

'I can't seem to find anything I do like when I look in the mirror. There are just fat bits everywhere: my arms, thighs, chin, arms, waist, bottom.'

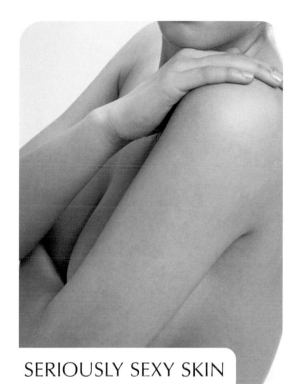

SERIOUSLY SEXY SKIN

Your skin is your largest organ. It not only holds all your bits in but is also a reflection of your inner health. Taking care of your skin should be as much of a habit as washing your hair and brushing your teeth. Follow the simple rules of cleanse, tone and moisturize and you're well on your way to glowing skin. And don't forget to protect your skin from the sun, pollution and cold: a moisturizer that contains a sun protection factor (SPF) of at least 15 is a must. Remember to wear sunscreen every day, even when it's cloudy, as sun rays will still get in and damage your skin. The result is premature ageing and wrinkles that will leave you looking older than you really are.

- If you're prone to dry skin, place a bowl of water next to the radiator in the winter months to absorb the dry heat. It'll stop your skin turning prune-like.
- Eat superfoods such as avocadoes, blueberries and salmon.
- Drink before you're thirsty. Water is the best beauty trick out there.
- Make sure you apply sunscreen to your hands too, as these are the first parts of your body to show signs of premature ageing.
- Keep a tube of hand cream next to your desk or in your bag and apply a few times a day to ward off dryness.
- Avoid dieting, especially crash dieting. If it makes you feel any better, remember that slightly plump people have fewer wrinkles than those who are stick-thin.
- Excessive alcohol consumption will cause your skin to dry out and fine spider-like veins may appear on your nose and cheeks.
- Sleep really is equal to a facelift. Get at least seven hours a night for a refreshed, youthful glow.

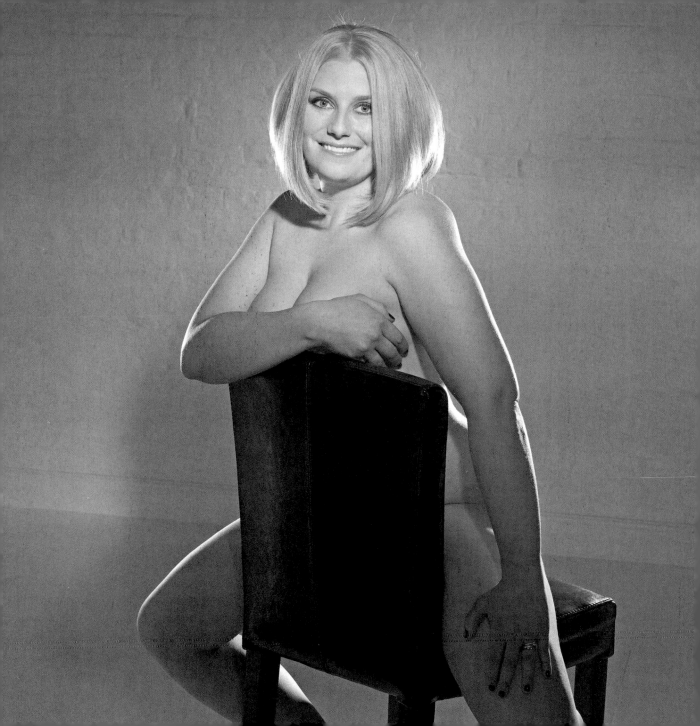

THE RESULT

With her magic knickers, fishnets and hot new haircut Liz felt ready for anything!

And the naked shot?

'It was very liberating to be able to pose nude in front of a roomful of people. I never thought I'd be able to do a naked photo shoot.'

'There's certainly a lot less shyness in the way I'm dressing now. And I'm not always undressing in secret with the lights off either. It's a very big step forward for me. I am trying to take a bit of time out after a shower to put some moisturizer on, which probably doesn't sound like much but for me it's quite a big change, because I never did anything like that in the past.'

'I definitely look good naked now. '

Flesh is fabulous. Bumpy, lumpy and funky. It's the number one wonder of the world.

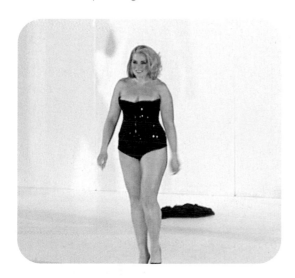

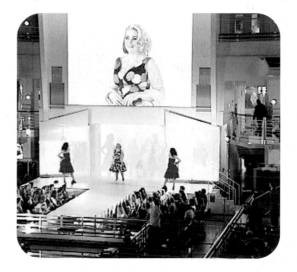

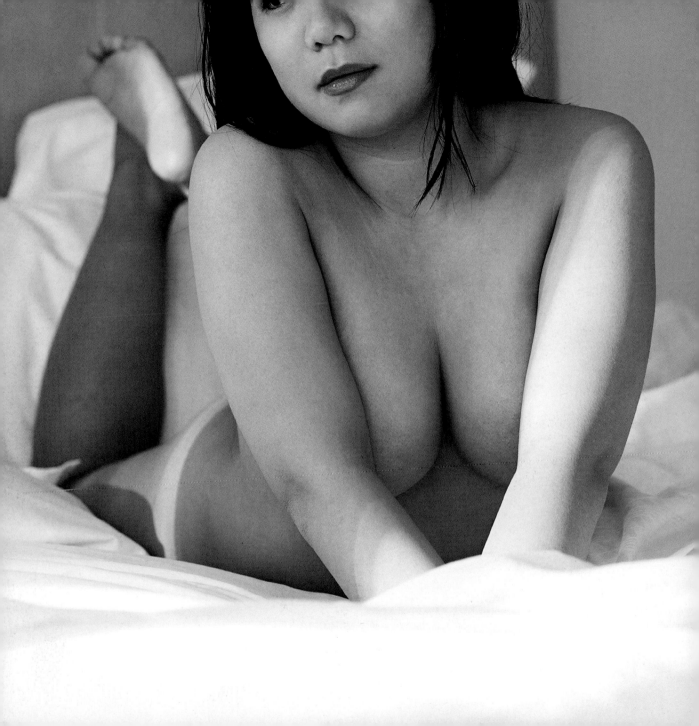

GETTING BACK IN THE SACK

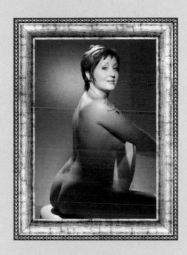

Leana Grech, 33, was a single mum from Wallington who felt she'd completely lost her sex appeal. Since becoming a mother she'd forgotten what it was like to be a woman and she hadn't had sex for four years. Leana had buried her sexy side for so long and had learnt to ignore her needs and desires. She was ashamed of her barrel-shape body and non-existent waist and covered it up in a wardrobe of unflattering clothes. Leana had a horror of communal changing rooms and when she did go shopping she cut the labels out of her clothes so that she didn't have to be reminded of her size.

We made it our mission to give Leana back the style and confidence she so desperately needed. First we showed her how to work her body to look good with her clothes on. Second, and more importantly, we showed her that it was possible to look good naked and feel confident with herself.

Even Leana's little boy Billy believed that his Mum could dress in a more girly way. 'I'd like to see Mummy in a beautiful Princess dress,' he said.

IN THE MIRROR

After four years of avoiding full-length mirrors, especially in front of other people, it was an emotional moment for Leana when she was confronted with her reflection. 'I'm just like a tree trunk – I have a tree trunk body that sits on a pair of legs,' she said. 'All I can see is fat: fat legs, fat stomach. I'm a big fat slug.' Leana would not contemplate letting anyone see her naked with the lights on.

She had a long way to go. What Leana didn't realize was that, like 98% of women in Britain who dislike their bodies, she has a beautiful face and figure but just didn't have the know-how or confidence to show her shape off to its best advantage.

It had been four years since Leana's last relationship and she was seriously out of practice. She genuinely feared that she might have forgotten what to do in the bedroom. If she was serious about getting some action, therefore, she needed to realize how gorgeous

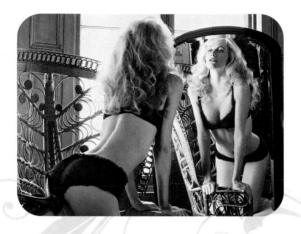

she was and leave the frumpy wardrobe far, far behind her.

'I've got bags of clothes in my wardrobe that don't fit me, because I never bother to try them on before buying. Once my little boy has gone to bed I just sort of sit around. I hardly ever go out,' she confessed.

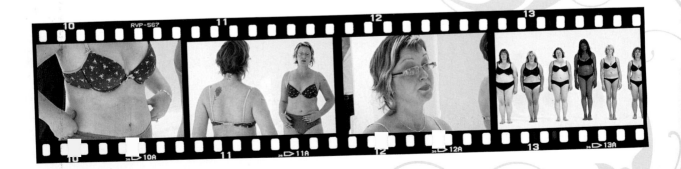

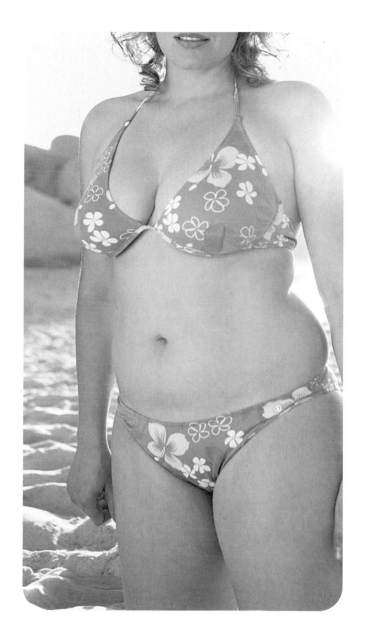

'When I look in the mirror I just see the woman I promised myself I'd never become.'

BODY PERCEPTION

With a 32-inch waist, Leana definitely had curves, but she had blinded herself to any positive parts of her body. In a line-up of women whose waists measured between 30 and 45-inches, she had the second smallest. But Leana's body image was so distorted that she thought that her waist was actually 41 inches. That's an extra nine inches. Even when confronted with her naked image Leana was still unable to see how svelte she really was. She had been dressing a figure that was an extraordinary two and a half stone heavier than it really was.

THE MAKEOVER

Leana had a typical apple-shaped body: no discernible shape from shoulders to hipbones, then thin and shapely legs. Up to 80% of British woman have an apple shape, or elements of the apple combined with other shapes. Most struggle with their wardrobe. And yet an apple silhouette is easy to dress in fashionable clothing – trapeze dresses over leggings, tights or skinny jeans are the apple's best friends. Once you've identified what parts of your body you want to accentuate and what you want to camouflage, shopping is a doddle.

Balance is the key when it comes to dressing apple-shaped figures – so your top-heavy shape won't topple over. We showed Leana how a trapeze-style dress (see opposite) would skim over her larger torso, but flaunt her fabulous pins. Add a belt and you've not only

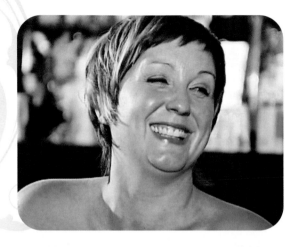

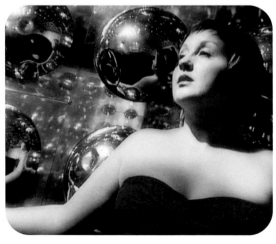

Up to 80% of British women have an apple shape, or elements of an apple combined with other shapes.

The Rules

APPLE SHAPES
Go for
- Wrap tops, which will emphasize your great boobs and create a waist.
- A correct-fitting bra.
- Trapeze or A-line dresses. These will skim over the largest part of your body and make your perfect pins look even longer and sexier.
- Flared or bootleg-cut trousers to balance your lower body with your upper.
- Materials such as chiffon and silk that will soften a bulkier upper body.
- Simple patterns.
- Belts to give a defined waist. A bold colour and eye-catching material will do even more to help separate your top half from your bottom.

Avoid
- Baggy or puff-sleeved tops. These will only make your shoulders and arms look bigger. Tailored tops are a better choice.
- Large or bold patterns that will emphasize your larger upper half.
- Ruffles and gathers which will just add width and weight.
- Tight bottoms that will make you look even larger on top.
- Trousers that have a front pleat, as these will only add inches to your waist and tummy.
- Pencil or tight-fitting skirts. The balance will be all wrong.

got a second wardrobe option, but an instant waspish-waist. Other ideal dress styles for apple body shapes are wraparounds and shift dresses. These show off your slim legs and emphasize your enviable rack. Look for jersey material too. With the right bump-smoothing pants, even clinging material is a possibility. A bra is especially important – apple shapes tends to have large boobs, so the bra that fits correctly will help support as well as create some much-needed shape. All without stepping foot inside a gym.

Apple shapes can do with some extra definition round their bum, so if you're going to wear jeans, look for designs that have pockets with flaps on the rear as these will add some sexy curves. Bootleg trousers or flared pants will also help to balance out a wider bust and shoulders.

We taught Leana that an apple body shape doesn't mean that she has to cover up from head to toe. With flattering and figure-enhancing underwear, she could choose to dress her apple shape, or even create a more timeless hourglass figure. It took a while, but eventually Leana realized that the only thing holding her back from being a sassy mama was her self-esteem and she felt confident enough to get out there and strut her stuff. She even managed to visit a changing room! 'I feel that every single woman should learn how to be confident naked,' Leana said. 'Women shouldn't be ashamed of their bodies or feel they have to hide them under clothes like I used to.'

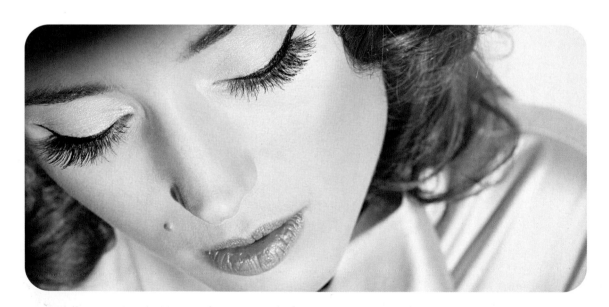

Salon Style

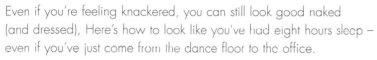

HOW TO LOOK GOOD KNACKERED

Even if you're feeling knackered, you can still look good naked
(and dressed), Here's how to look like you've had eight hours sleep –
even if you've just come from the dance floor to the office.

Step one

Remove any old make-up from around the eyes and then spritz the face and body with a water spritzer. This plumps up the skin and creates a smoother, more even surface on which to apply your tinted moisturizer.

Step two

Apply an eye concealer or brightener under the eye to lift any dark areas (see box p.43). Use your ring finger as this will prevent dragging (which could create premature wrinkles).

Step three

Use a lilac eye shadow on the lid. This freshens the skin and brightens the whites of the eyes. Avoid anything too pink or lurid when you're tired

Step four

Finish the eyes with lashings of false lash-effect mascara. Only apply to the top lashes after you've curled them.

Step five

Add some colour to the cheeks. Choose a peachy shade if you are blonde or fair and a pinker shade if you are a brunette or have a warmer skin tone.

Step six

Warm up dull, tired skin by moisturizing with a bronzing product. Apply to the apples of your cheeks, your chin and your forehead – everywhere the sun tans you.

Step seven

Rev up the skin by brushing on a loose bronzer after you've moisturized. Run it up the backs of your legs to create the illusion of skyscraper pins.

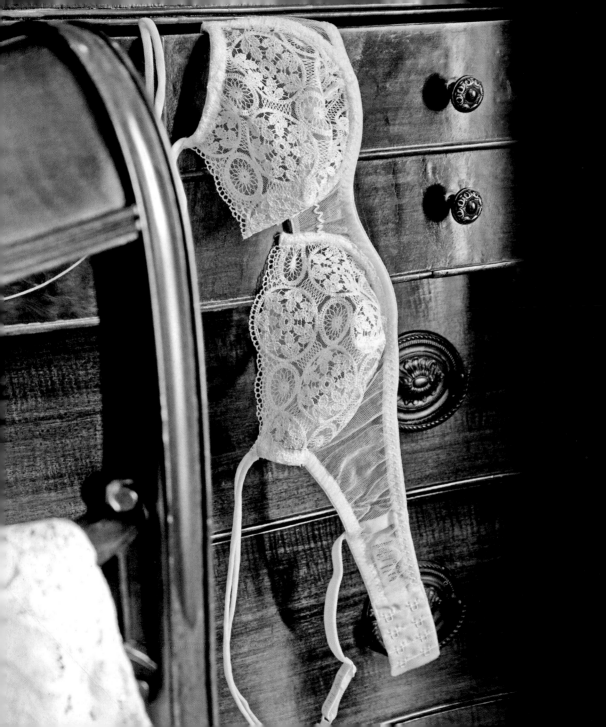

FROM FLAB TO FAB

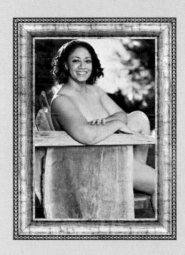

Rock chicks never die, they just move to Crawley. Cindy Bristow had hit the big Four-O, and was feeling as if the best years of her life – and her figure – were now behind her. As a mum of three children and wife to Dan, Cindy really had it all, but could only see what she no longer had: her youth, her freedom and her 20-year-old body.

An extra burden for Cindy was her gorgeous husband's age: Dan was nine years younger than Cindy, which meant that she put pressure on herself to look younger than her years. This created some tension in their relationship, as Cindy constantly compared her body to the one she used to have. Cindy believed that Dan was disappointed whenever he saw her naked, so refused to let him see her in the buff.

Let's face it, after three children your body is never going to be the same, no matter how much time you spend in the gym. But there's no reason why other people need to know that you've got a baby belly and stretch marks. Looking good is about feeling good, which begins with your wardrobe…

WHAT SHE SAW

Like so many of you out there, Cindy dressed in the classic uniform of the body loather – baggy, shapeless jumpers and sweatshirts. She described her aim as 'blending into the background' and herself as 'your average tired, busy mum'. Cindy didn't realise that her wardrobe choices actually made her look much larger and frumpier than she really was.

Cindy became tearful when she faced herself in the mirror. 'My body is an embarrassment to me,' she said. 'The confidence I had before I my children has completely disappeared. I have two tummies rather than one and my body is like a squeezy toy. Someone has squeezed it in the middle and it's just stayed out of proportion.'

Dan had done what he could, but his comments had fallen on deaf ears. 'I try to reassure Cindy that she has a great body, but she can't take any compliments at all,' said Dan. Cindy hated Dan touching her stomach, which made bedroom action somewhat difficult!

Instead of looking back and longing for the lifestyle and body shape of her younger self, Cindy needed to come to terms with her figure and learn how to dress her shape. Most of all, she had to love herself again: lumps, bumps and all. 'When I look in the mirror it's not me I see, not the confident person that I've always been,' she said. If you feel alienated from your body, you will never look or feel good.

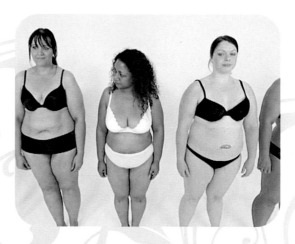

BODY PERCEPTION

Cindy's body image had certainly got the better of her. In a line-up of women she placed her tummy measurement two and half inches larger than it was. Yet deep down she knew what the problem was. When we asked her what the difference was between her and one of our other line-up lovelies she was spot on: confidence.

We were determined to expose Cindy to her naked self until she was forced to accept it. A drive through her home town of Crawley in a van plastered with her undressed image was brutal but necessary. Vans honked their horns and passers-by gave the thumbs-up. At first she was horribly embarrassed, but soon it dawned on her that not everybody could be wrong.

THE MAKEOVER

Cindy's best assets were her endless legs, even though she believed they were riddled with cellulite, and were too short and too fat. Her boobs were in pretty good shape too. Body confidence is all about concentrating on and highlighting your best bits and hiding the bits you aren't so happy about. Once Cindy realized that her curves were not for hiding away, we were able to make the most of them with some lessons in style.

We chose a streamlined, fitted jacket for Cindy, teamed with a wide, figure-hugging belt. This accentuated her luscious boobs and hips. A well-structured jacket is every woman's best friend. Team it with straight-legged, dark trousers and you'll immediately look years younger. Underneath was another of Cindy's new secrets – a sexy, figure-hugging basque.

For nights out on the town with Dan, a hot pink spotted dress, with a wide band at the waist, created the illusion of a perfect hourglass figure, without an extra inch of fat. Cindy was lucky – her lovely chocolate-coloured skin can cope with intense, vibrant colours. By vamping up her boobs and showing off her perfect pins, Cindy discovered that nobody, least of all her, was paying attention to her supposedly jelly-belly.

If, like Cindy, you've got a wobbly tum, don't despair. Instead, hold it in with stomach control pants and wide-belts. You'll turn your worst bit into your sexiest bit in no time at all.

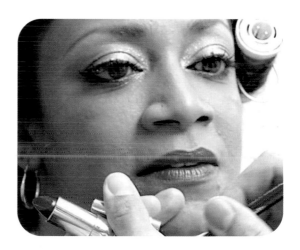

'I have two tummies rather than one and my body is like a squeezy toy.'

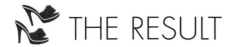

THE RESULT

For her naked photo shoot, we whisked Cindy away to a wonderful countryside setting so she could truly get back to nature! Cindy's mane was trimmed, shaped and given a lot more bounce, which perfectly finished off her look. 'I can't believe I just did that,' she confessed. After that, and some lessons in serious strutting, the catwalk was a piece of cake.

Salon Style

QUICK MANICURE AND PEDICURE

Massage a good cuticle oil into your nails to soften the skin.

Shape your fingernails with a fine nail file, using a 'side to middle' movement. Never file your nail backwards and forwards as this weakens the nail. The ideal natural shape for a fingernail is a mirror of the shape of the cuticle. For toenails, this should be straight across so that the nail is square.

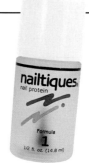

Gently scrape the base of the nail with a cuticle trimmer to remove the thin layer of skin that sticks to the nail plate. Gently lift away any remaining skin at the base of the nail.

Buff the nails to give them a healthy shine.

Remove any remaining debris from the surface of the nail and clean under the edge with disposable orange stick (a bit like a giant tooth pick).

Apply a strengthening nail formula either before or after your nail polish, although some look fine worn on their own.

Finish with a good moisturizer specifically formulated for hands and feet. For an extra-strength moisturizing treatment, apply the cream, then put on some gloves and socks and leave overnight.

86% of women think their tummy is their least sexy area

Cindy had come a very long way in the space of just six weeks. There wasn't a trace of the unconfident, tearful Mum who hid behind baggy jumpers every day. On the catwalk, with her fantastic makeover, she held her head up high and really strutted her stuff. At last Cindy understood what Dan had been telling her: she really was one hot Mama!

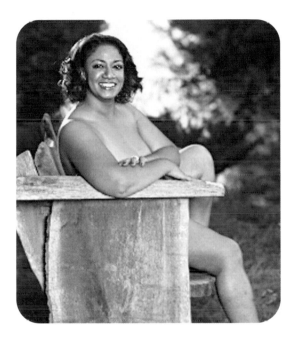

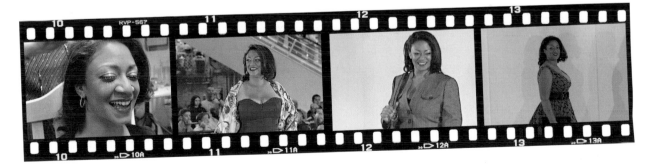

Skirts

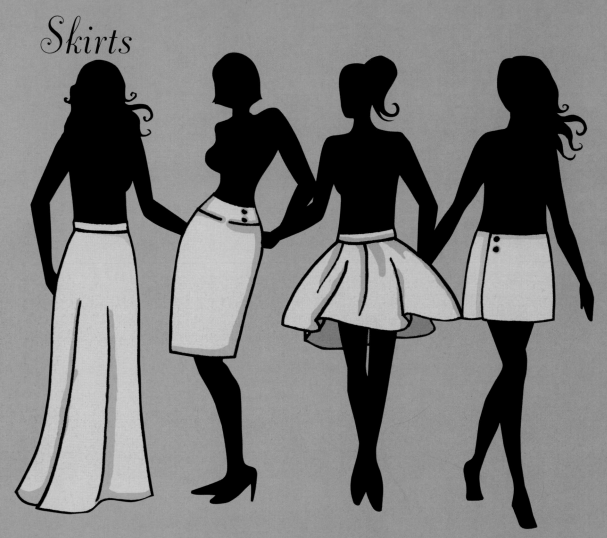

FULL
FEATURES: floor-length with acres of material
GOOD FOR: tall, willowy types
BAD FOR: petite

STRAIGHT
FEATURES: as the name implies
GOOD FOR: hourglass
BAD FOR: apple, pencil

BALLERINA
FEATURES: sits wide on the hips
GOOD FOR: straight up-and-down figures
BAD FOR: apple

MINI
FEATURES: cut high on the thigh
GOOD FOR: anybody under 30, long-legged lovelies
BAD FOR: pear, hourglass

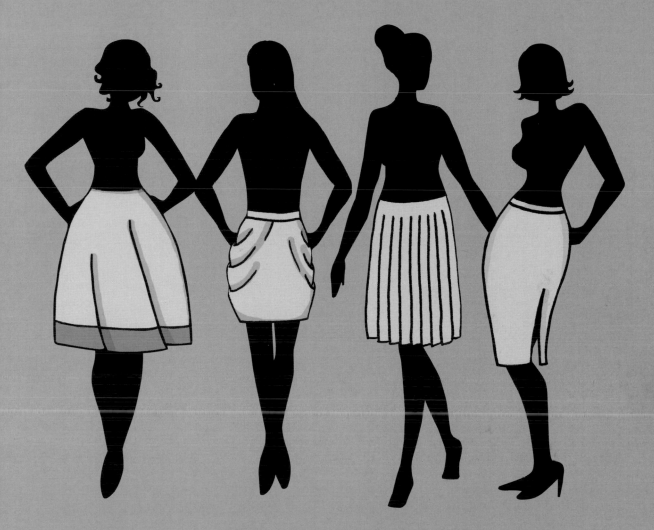

A-LINE

FEATURES: flares from the waist
GOOD FOR: pear, hourglass
BAD FOR: apple

TULIP

FEATURES: shaped like
the flower!
GOOD FOR: straight up-and-
down figures
BAD FOR: pear

PLEATED

FEATURES: has either skinny or
wide folds
GOOD FOR: all body shapes
BAD FOR: pot bellies (a wide waistband solves this)

PENCIL

FEATURES: figure-hugging
with a slit
GOOD FOR: hourglass
BAD FOR: pear

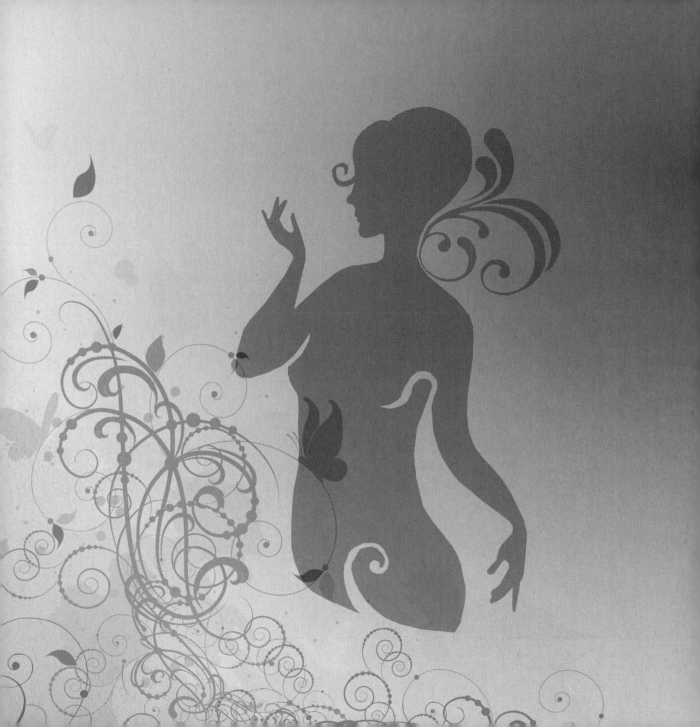

Chapter 4

BUM WRAP

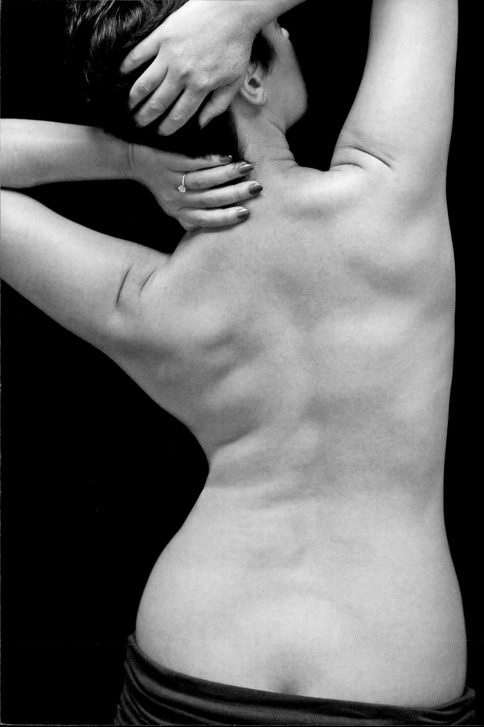

DOES MY BUM LOOK BIG IN THIS?

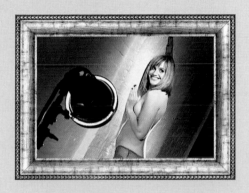

Becky Newman's nickname for herself – Becky Big Bum – perfectly summed up her perception of her body. This mum of one did everything she possibly could to avoid having to look at her posterior – wearing long, shapeless, woolly jumpers and hiding in the bathroom to dress. Becky drove her partner, Mark, to despair by constantly asking whether her 'bum looked big in this'. The truth was, Mark would rarely get the opportunity to see her bottom anyway! The pair were lucky to have the sea right on their doorstep, but getting Becky into her bikini was a non-starter.

While Becky made jokes about the size of her derriere to friends and family, this was just a façade – the fact was, it made her truly miserable. Even though she had a typical size 12 bottom, there was no convincing Becky that her baggy clothes and dowdy denim were actually making her bum look larger than it really was.

Our mission was to get Becky out of those shapeless sacks, and into some flattering, bottom-baring bikinis.

WHAT SHE SAW

Becky approached mirrors with great trepidation. 'If I jump up and down my cheeks slap together – it's like I'm giving myself a round of applause!' she said. And she confessed that the size of her bum had been an issue for her since she was a teenager.

Two out of three British women are pear-shaped, which means they are around one size larger on their bottom than they are on their top. So it's more usual to be this shape than any other body shape. But Becky thought that she was a unique case. She was a slight pear, but her perception was so skewed that she believed her bum to be four inches larger than it was. Until Becky accepted the size of her bottom, there was no point in teaching her how to dress. We enlisted the help of some passers-by, who gave us positive comments.

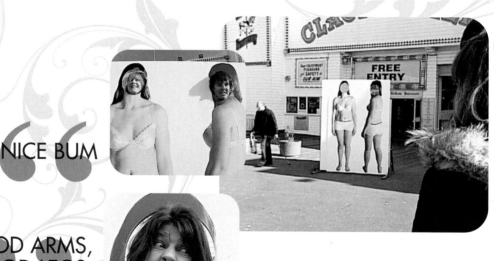

"NICE BUM

GOOD ARMS, GOOD LEGS, VERY SEXY

I'D LIKE TO HAVE A BODY LIKE THAT

'Everybody tells me to stop worrying about my bum and I've tried, but it's all I see.'

Covering up her bottom with long tops and jumpers tied around her waist actually drew attention to Becky's rear, not away from it. This is a mistake that many women make. If you want to slim down an area, reduce the amount of material covering it: remember, less is more.

Time to fix Becky's bum dress sense…

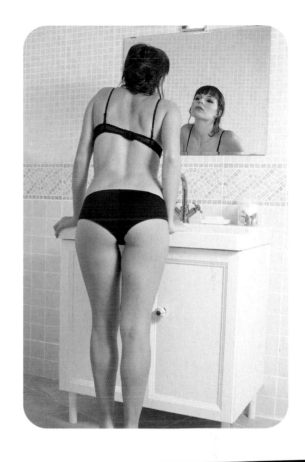

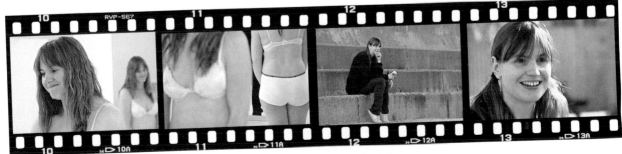

THE MAKEOVER

To draw attention away from Becky's bottom, we dressed her in an Empire-line dress with a defined and detailed line, which showed off her slender shoulders and pert boobs, while skimming over her much-hated bottom. Heels were added, as they are a must to lengthen the distance between the floor and hips. 'I seem to be getting thinner by the minute – with every outfit,' she said. As Becky's confidence grew, she began to accept her real shape for what it really was.

SUMMER DRESS RULES

The summer dress is the most versatile item you'll every buy. It'll take you from the bedroom to the beach to the bar. When choosing your summer dress pay particular attention to the neckline as this will help you decide if the shape is right for you.

- Pear shape: empire line dresses that end above the knee are ideal. The neckline tends to sit just across the boobs.
- Apple shape: V-necklines flatter your upper chest and make your neck look slimmer and longer.
- Pencil shape: diagonal dresses will create curvy interest.
- Sloping shoulders: strapless dresses will make your shoulders seem more pronounced and defined.

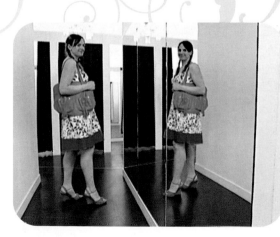

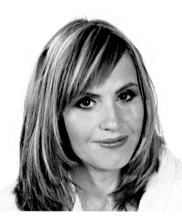

Salon Style

HOW TO FAKE TAN

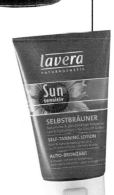

We all know that sunning ourselves is bad: bad for the skin, bad for the wrinkles and bad for our health. So how should a beach babe get that golden glow? After all, a tan helps to make you appear thinner, healthier and more toned. The secret, girls, is to fake it. Here's how:

Step One

Have a shower, but don't use any perfumed soaps or body washes. If you do use these, then leave your skin for half an hour before applying your tan.

Step Two

Exfoliate, exfoliate, exfoliate. Sloughing off dead skin will give you a nice blank canvas on which to apply your 'paint'. Use a body scrub with granules to get a lovely, smooth finish.

Step Three

Dry your skin thoroughly. If you have them, wear gloves. This will stop the mixture staining your skin and giving your tanning secret away.

Step Four

Then, beginning at your feet, apply your tan. Use firm, even strokes over your main body, but lighter strokes over your joints, such as elbows and knees, so that you don't use too much mixture on these dryer areas.

Step Five

If you don't have a separate face-tanning product, dilute your body tanner with some moisturizer. Pull you hair back from your face and blend the tanner up into your hairline, but not too far, otherwise it can appear orange.

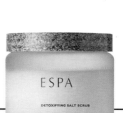

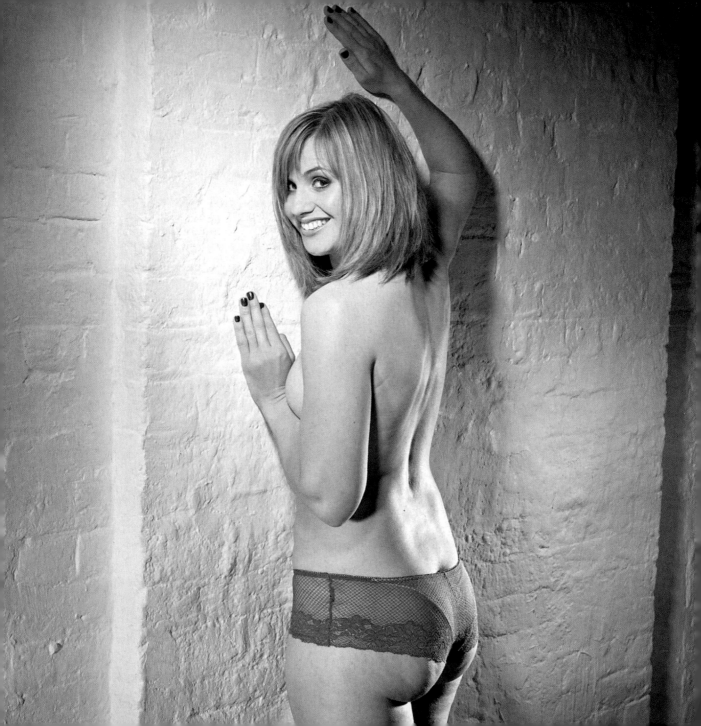

THE RESULT

In just six weeks we had managed to persuade Becky to transform her attitude to her body. She was taking more care of herself, particularly her bottom area, by exercising regularly to tone up her rear. What's more, she had begun undressing in front of her husband again. She had cleared her wardrobe of dark, bum-hiding jumpers and had hit the high street to sort out her summer wardrobe with some fabulous flouncy frocks.

For her naked photo session Becky was buffed, bronzed and blow-dried – she looked so beautiful!

Even the former 'Becky Big Bum' seemed to finally get it. 'I'm quite proud of myself,' she said. 'Damn I look good naked!'

White outfits can make you look bigger, unless you know how to wear them. Add a belt in a dark or metallic colour.

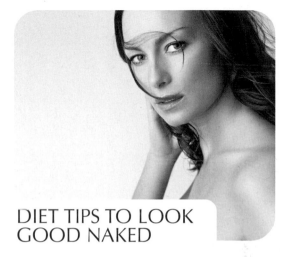

DIET TIPS TO LOOK GOOD NAKED

If you want to eliminate bloating, excess water retention and rid yourself of that muffin top, here are some simple steps you can take.

- Avoid salty foods. Cut out white foods for one week. This includes white bread, pasta, potatoes, sugar and dairy. It's tough, but it'll be worth it.

- Ban the booze. Alcohol is a no-no if you want to lose weight. It's full of 'empty' calories, which means calories that have no nutritional gain. Your body has no option but to store these as fat.

- Think raw. Foods that are closest to their raw states are fabulous foods. Fruit, vegetables and nuts are all filling, but love your body.

- Drink drink drink. Water that is. At least two litres a day. It'll stop you feeling hungry and flush out those nasty toxins.

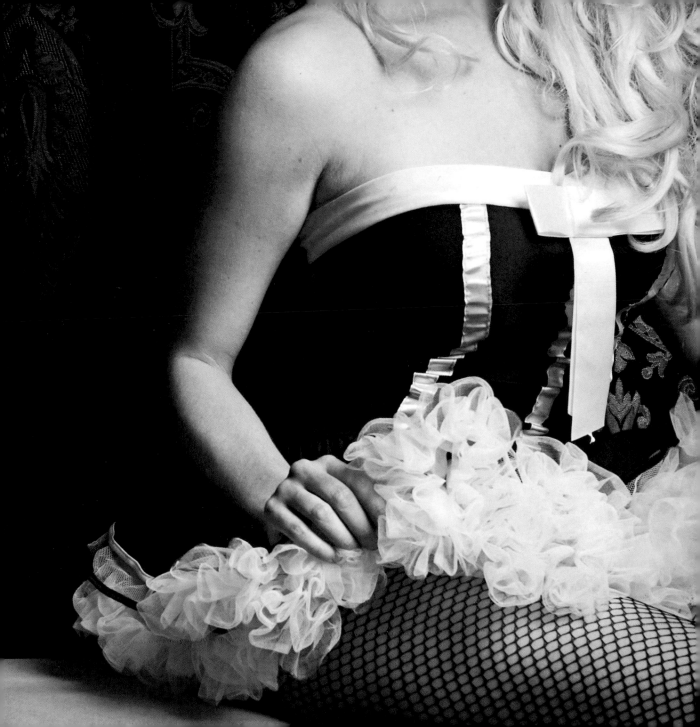

SMALL
BUT PERFECTLY FORMED

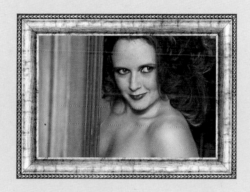

Ali Birch, 25, was engaged to be married, but was so self-conscious about her body that she had postponed her wedding to fiancé Matt. Perfectly formed at a petite 4 feet 10 inches, Ali felt that her little girl complex was beginning to affect other parts of her life. Even though 6-footer Matt had fancied her from the moment he saw her, Ali preferred to dress in kids' pyjamas than flaunt her figure in front of him. While he would be out on a Saturday night, Ali would stay at home with just the dog and the telly for company.

Ali just couldn't see the gorgeous redhead who, according to Matt, 'had the height of Kylie, the body of Jennifer Ellison and the face of the model Lily Cole'. Instead she felt, and dressed, like a child. And ever since her childhood Ali had believed that she was fat, a belief she had carried with her through adulthood. Her thighs were particular objects of hatred. We had to deal with this 'child complex' before Ali could dress like, and become, the sexy woman she clearly had the potential to be.

IN THE MIRROR

'When I look in the mirror at my body I'm disgusted. Quite often I'll stand in front of the mirror and cry. Because I hate the way I look. I hate my thighs and I hate my wobbly tummy.'

Ali's biggest hang-up was her thighs. And yet Ali's thigh measurement, at 22½ inches, was below the national average of 24 inches. This didn't wash with her, however. 'My thighs look like chicken drumsticks,' she said.

Ali felt that when she went out to a public place she was being looked at and laughed at. Her body image was crippling her self-esteem and we urgently had to tell her that she was a gorgeous young woman – and then help her to believe it.

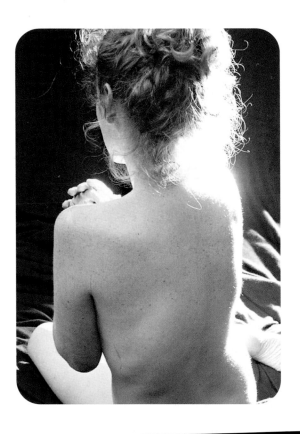

'Quite often I'll stand in front of the mirror and cry.'

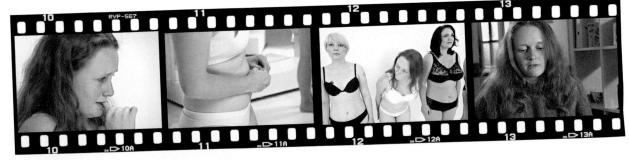

THE MAKEOVER

Ali hadn't always believed that she was a lost cause. In fact, she had paintings hanging throughout her house of the woman she wanted to be. What Ali hadn't realized was that she already was the woman in the paintings. But even more beautiful. Ali's tiny hourglass frame could carry off most looks, but she had to steer away from the children's department and shop with the grown ups.

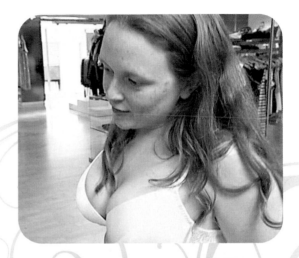

For Ali's wardrobe makeover we went for a pair of skinny jeans teamed with a looser-fitting top in this season's vibrant purple. Skinny jeans have been all the rage and they seem set to stay. But you don't have to be Kate Moss-skinny to wear them – the secret is choosing the right pair and teaming them with the right top.

Ali thought that she was far too short and plump to successfully wear skinnies, but her petite measurements were actually just right. Always choose a pair slightly too long for you – teamed with high heels they'll make your legs look endless. We chose a pair of wicked purple heels that catapulted Ali into a sexy, gorgeous woman.

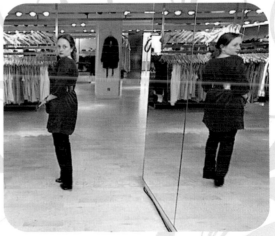

One negative effect of skinny jeans is the creation of a 'muffin top' – the excess skin that hangs over either side of your waistband. To counteract this, either wear your jeans with magic knickers to hold you in, or team your tight-fitting jeans with a looser, A-line top that skims your lumps and bumps.

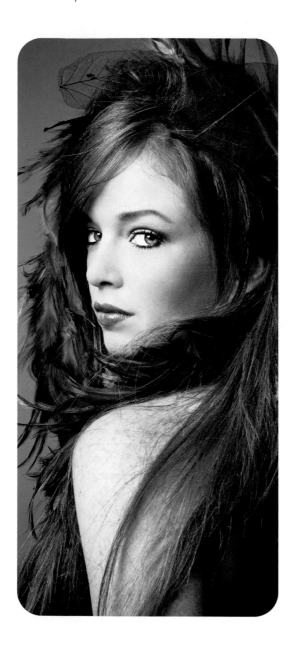

We finished off Ali's outfit with a great waist-cinching belt. Whenever dressing in the latest colours or fashions, make sure that you're always showing off your best assets – in Ali's case, her killer waistline.

'I'm feeling a lot better about my body. I wouldn't say that I love it yet, but I'm certainly starting to feel more comfortable in my own skin,' she said. Ali joined a gym and in just four weeks had lost an inch and a half off her waist and half an inch off each thigh. Her positive body image didn't stop there. She also began eating more healthily and things had begun hotting up in the bedroom too. 'Our sex life was pants, but now it's panties,' said fiancé Matt.

REDHEAD RULES

If you've been blessed with a fiery mane, then you know that your hair is the most eye-catching thing you can wear. So be careful not to overpower it. Instead wear colours that complement your hair and skin tone. White, black and green all provide a base on to which you can add some gold, copper or jewelled accessories. Avoid wearing pink on top if your complexion is slightly pink too – but if you have a true peaches-and-cream skin tone, then a soft pink is extremely flattering. Remember: the warmer your skin tone and hair colour, the warmer the colour you can wear. And the same works for paler shades too.

The Rules

PETITE SHAPES

If you're under 5 foot 4 inches, then you're classified as a 'petite'. It may sound cute and delicate, but if you get the proportions wrong you can end up looking shorter and wider than you really are. The trick is to highlight your best area, whether it's your slender legs, tiny waist or curvy bum, and camouflage the rest.

Go for

- A good seamstress. Fitted clothes will make the most of your figure while baggy clothes will not only make you look shapeless, but shorter and more squat too.
- Bright colours. But stick to just the one.
- Small prints. These will make you look taller.
- Tops that finish just above your waistline will make your legs appear longer. The same goes for jackets – choose one where the waistline nips in slightly above your natural waist.
- Slip dresses or empire lines, to elongate your legs.
- Pencil skirts will give you some seriously sexy curves. You can can get away with mini skirts too.

Avoid

- Belts. These will make your body look smaller, as they will break up your appearance into two pieces.
- Batwing or loose, flowing sleeves. Cap or short sleeves are best.
- Cropped jeans or trousers. These will do nothing to lengthen your legs.
- Chunky accessories and large bags. They will simply overwhelm your frame.

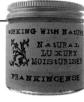

Salon Style

FACE MASKS

Taking time to treat yourself to some serious pampering will pay immediate dividends, and one of the best ways you can do is to apply a good-quality face mask. You'll immediately look and feel better and your skin will thank you over and over again, with fewer spots, softer lines and glowing cheeks.

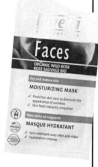

Step One

Cleanse your face thoroughly with warm water.

Step Two

Pat dry and apply your chosen face mask. If you have oily skin, choose a mask that dries out; if you have dry skin, a mask that remains moist is preferable.

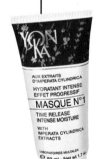

Step Three

Leave for the length of time indicated on the packet – relax in a bath, or read your favourite magazine.

Step Four

Remove the mask by applying a warm face or muslin cloth to your skin. It's important you don't drag your skin down but instead sweep the mask away with gentle upward movements. Continue until all traces of the mask have been removed. Finish by splashing with cold water.

Step Five

To truly get the best out of your face mask routine, finish by applying a serum, followed by your normal moisturizer and eye cream. If you have applied the mask just before bedtime, use a night cream.

THE RESULT

With her gorgeous figure and distinctive colouring, Ali was finally turning heads and drawing attention to herself, instead of hiding away at home. Her new, darker tone of red made her more bed head than sleepy head and turned Ali into a sexy, beautiful woman. Six weeks ago, Ali wouldn't even undress in front of her husband to be. Just a short time later she bared all in a naked photo shoot. 'I'm not a little girl anymore. I felt curvy, womanly and amazing. I loved it.'

Ali's final challenge was to strut down the runway in her lingerie, even though she was terrified of letting others see her body, especially her thighs and bottom. But the pocket Venus summoned up the courage to do just that. No more shy little girl – there was no holding her back this time.

'She looked superb and I think she now finally realizes what I see when I look at her,' said Matt.

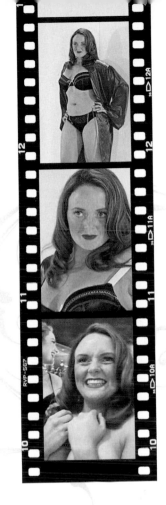

Women in the UK obsess about their bodies every 15 minutes.

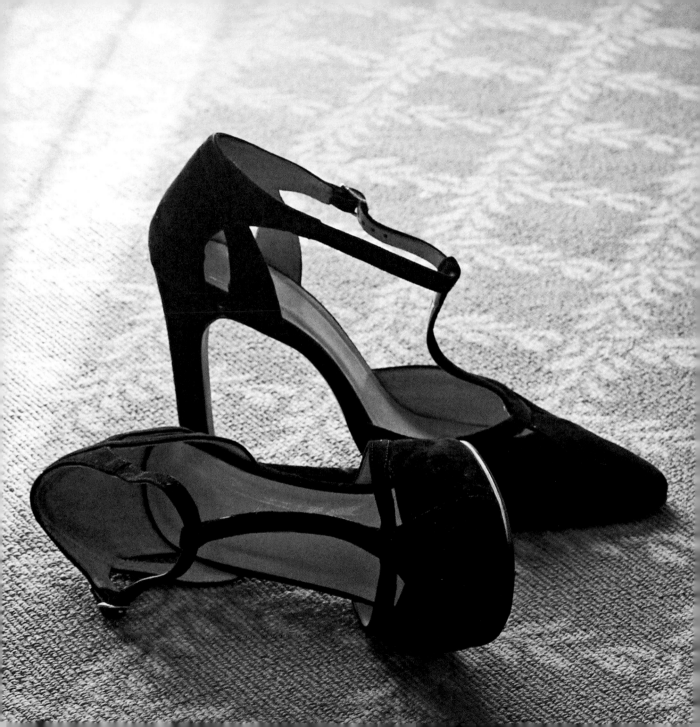

RUNWAY GODDESS

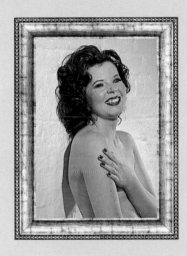

Leanne Townsend, 27, was trapped in a cycle of 'ugly days'. She loathed her legs and couldn't see what everybody else could: that she had a gorgeous, womanly figure.

Leanne did everything she could to camouflage her legs, even wearing tights on hot summer days. Her husband Lee hadn't seen her naked for more than five years, even though he showered her with compliments and admiration. He bought her sexy lingerie, to no avail. Leanne hid it under piles of tights in her room. If they had sex she would wear special tights, so that Lee still couldn't see her. Leanne shied away from affection, and told Lee that she was busy or that he was interrupting her if he tried to kiss or hug her.

'I married Leanne for who she is, not for her legs,' said Lee. 'And the crazy thing is, she has great legs! Really sexy!'

Leanne slobbed around in tracksuit pants and baggy trousers, which did nothing to emphasize her shape. We had to convince Leanne that she was missing out on her life by hiding her legs, and herself, away and encourage her to get out there and start living – feet first!

IN THE MIRROR

It was a huge battle to get Leanne out of those tights. Then the confrontation with the glass was an even bigger battle. But only by peeling off those tights could we help Leanne peel away the negative preconceptions about herself.

'I think that my hips are huge; I've got stretch marks and scars. I don't feel like an attractive woman. I don't want to wear tights, but I have to wear them,' she said.

In a line-up of women whose thigh width measured from 22 to 27 inches, Leanne placed herself at the mid-way point. In other words, she added another six inches to her thigh measurement. The truth was, she had an enviable slim figure, and that included her legs. When we took her out on the street and asked people to comment on her shape, the main reaction was that you just couldn't see it.

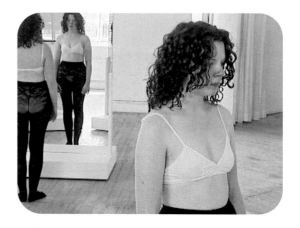

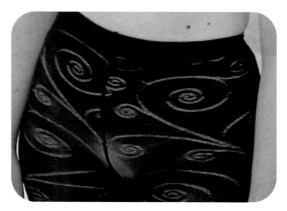

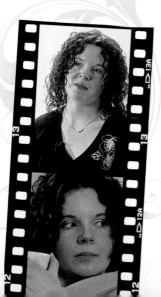

'My bum starts before my legs can finish.'

THE MAKEOVER

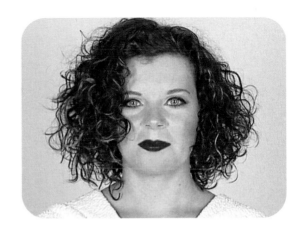

Leanne not only lived in her tights, she also wore another layer by constantly wearing her dressing gown when she was at home. 'If somebody came to the house at 4pm I'd have my dressing gown on,' she said. It was time to get rid of Leanne's old body image, layer by layer.

First step was to rid Leanne's wardrobe of her terrible tights and big pants and get her

Layering Rules

Layering isn't about piling items of clothing on top of each other until you resemble the Michelin man. Rather, it's a very clever way to create shape, curve and interest: although it's actually one of the hardest looks to get right. The key is to use clothing that fits and that complements the piece underneath it. So team a V-neck cardigan with a V-neck vest or shirt and a knee-length skirt with a knee-length jacket. Remember, you can layer clothing even on the warmest days using thin knits, camisoles or tank tops.

- Hourglass: this feminine shape suits most type of layers. A jacket that ends just above the hipline is ideal and should match the hemlines on your other layers.
- Pear: choose layers that will elongate the neckline. Try a form-fitting camisole or tank top under a well-structured jacket. Make certain that the jacket buttons sit around the largest part of your frame, and that the shoulder seams sit at your shoulders. If the jacket is too tight, it will simply accentuate bulk.
- Apple: create curves and balance with layering. Top a camisole with a thin-knitted top, with a deep V-neck. The V-shape of the jumper or cardigan will create a longer neck for you, while creating the illusion of a bust and small waist. Your camisole can peek out from under the cardigan.
- Tall and thin: use bulk to create a feminine, curvy look. Layer a large knit over a tank top, then add a wide belt to emphasize your waist. The colour of the tank should complement that of the large knit.

into figure-flattering underwear. She had so many wonderfully sexy smalls to choose from with that constant showering of gifts from her adoring husband. Once the basics were sorted, it was time to dress Leanne in outfits that flattered her legs.

We chose a halter-neck top, which flattered Leanne's small bust and made her shoulders look wider, an easy way to balance out the hips. Teamed with knee-length leggings,

Leanne could still feel like she was covered, although she was flashing more flesh than she had done in years. Heels were key, and we chose a killer pair for Leanne. Unless you have really skinny ankles, you should avoid ankle straps, as they just cut your leg in half.

After a top-to-toe treatment, including a pedicure, body polish and foot massage, Leanne also did her bit by joining a gym and started working out for the first time in years.

Salon Style

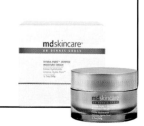

NIGHT CREAMS TO THE TEST

We spend around £48 million a year on night cream, so make sure you use yours correctly to help achieve that look of eternal youth.

How to prepare your skin at night

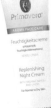

Using a muslin cloth or facecloth, wet your face with warm, NOT hot, water. Rub a dollop of cleanser between your hands and apply to your face. Spread the cream over your face using an upward movement. Use your cloth to remove the cream, but don't drag your skin. Then apply your night cream, again using upward movements, towards your hairline. Tap the cream, or a separate eye cream, around your eye using your ring finger (imagine that you're playing the piano). Now you're ready for your beauty sleep!

Choosing the right cream for you

Dry skin: look for products that contain essential fatty acids and oils such as rosehip and argon.

Oily skin: a lighter, water-based cream is best.

Normal skin: you're lucky – you can use any type of cream.

HOW TO TAKE ATTENTION AWAY FROM YOUR LEGS

Do

- Wear leggings if you don't feel comfortable showing off your entire leg. Aim for just below your knee, otherwise they'll crop you off and make you look shorter.

- Wear A-line dresses, to stop you from looking too small on top.

- Choose smocked or pin-tucked dresses which hug your waist and give the illusion of the perfect hourglass.

- Learn to love waistcoats. These will draw even more attention to your upper half and accentuate your waist.

- Wear high heels that elongate your legs. Go for as high as you can bear.

- Choose boots with a decent heel – these can be your best friend if you are uncomfortable with your legs. You'll look sexy, but you'll be covered.

- Wear knee-length dresses. These will hide your thighs and suggest that your legs are thin the entire way up from the ankle.

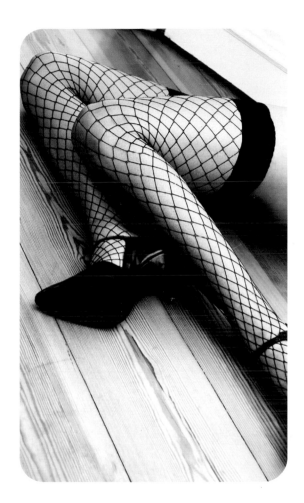

Don't

- Wear flats. The area between the floor and your hips should be as long as possible.

- Wear dresses or tops with thin straps. This will just make your shoulders look smaller and, therefore, your hips even wider.

- Forget to add a belt if you feel that you're looking a bit hip heavy.

- Wear shoes with an ankle strap. These will cut your legs off and make your ankles look heavier.

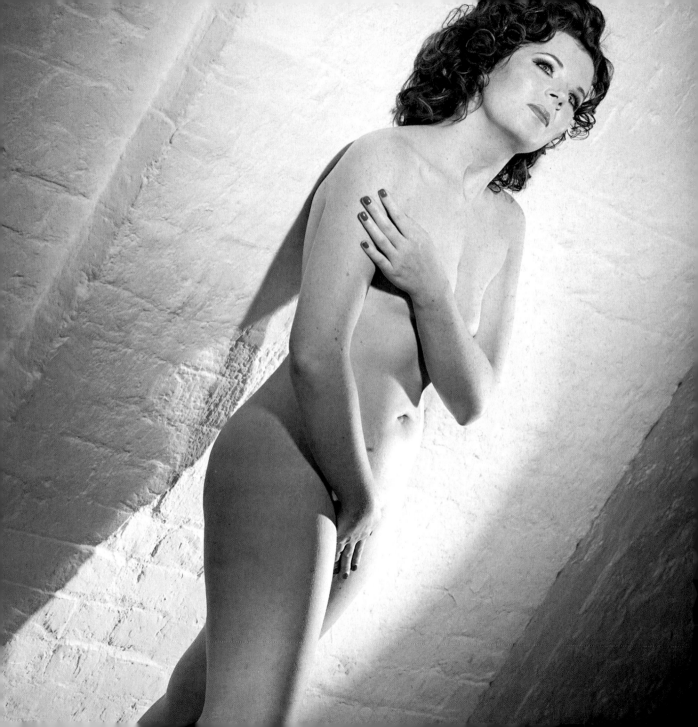

THE RESULT

Leanne had wonderful curly red hair but instead of making the most of this natural asset, she tried to tame her curls. We cut her hair into layers to emphasize her natural wave and gave her fire-engine red lips and nails to match her new exuberant, confident personality. After just six weeks, Leanne had gone from body loathing to body loving. Finally, when she looked in the mirror, she could honestly say that she liked what she saw. Finally, she could get out of those tights. What's more, her relationship with Lee was better than ever – she described it as 'like being married all over again'. And she was ready to strip off and take the plunge on the catwalk.

'I never thought in a million years that I would get my photograph taken naked. I feel liberated and that I can do anything.'

65% of women believe that their life would improve if they had a better body

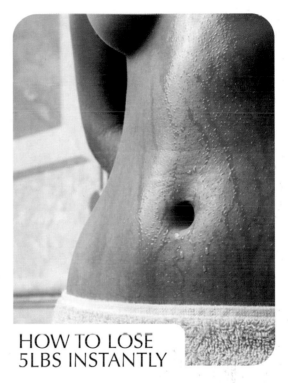

HOW TO LOSE 5LBS INSTANTLY

Pull your shoulders back, pull your tummy in. tuck your bottom under and hold your chin up high. Voila! You immediately look thinner, taller and, best of all, more confident.

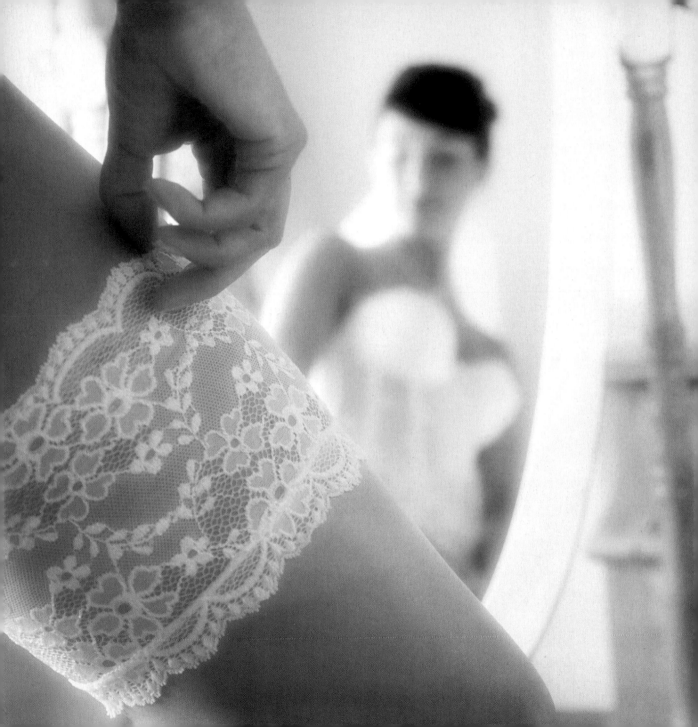

FROM BOUNCER TO BABE

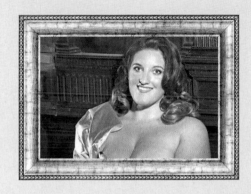

Ally Howard, 26, was stuck in a fashion and lifestyle contradiction. Working as a nanny by day and a nightclub bouncer by night meant that she was leading two very different lives – both sartorially and personally.

Ally had lost a lot of confidence and hadn't looked in the mirror for three years. She felt particularly lost when it came to dressing her body shape out of hours. In this she is not alone. It's a common problem for many women, who feel unsure when it comes to taking off their work 'uniform'. It's not about slobbing about in tracksuits – although these do have their place! Dressing off duty is all about wearing comfortable, soft and feminine clothes that express your personality. Ally's wardrobe was full of frumpy, baggy clothes that said nothing about who she was and everything about hiding her figure.

We set about getting Ally's off-duty outfit sorted, before teaching her how to put on the glitz. Ally had never had a boyfriend, so had no confidence in her sexuality or femininity. Our aim was to show her what a little sex kitten she really was.

IN THE MIRROR

Undressing in front of a mirror was a nightmare come true for Ally. She certainly didn't like what she saw. 'It's disgusting. I'm disgusting,' she said. 'A woman's figure is meant to be shapely and hourglass. I'm just a pear on legs.' Ally hated her tum and bum the most. Even though she knew she should try to lose weight and exercise, she despised her body so much that it was easier to just not think of her body as part of her.

Working as a bouncer meant she had to cultivate a hard shell – to appear tough and firm, not girly and giggly. She'd buried her feminine side so deep that even when she wasn't working she appeared strong and unapproachable.

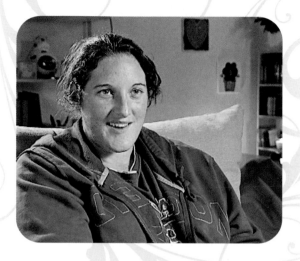

BODY PERCEPTION

Ally's main body problem was that she thought she had a huge bum – but it was all in her mind. In a line-up of women whose posteriors ranged from 46 to 51 inches, Ally judged her bottom as the biggest, when it was actually the smallest.

'I'm gobsmacked – absolutely gobsmacked.' Ally agreed that all the women in the line-up had gorgeous bums. It began to dawn on her that perhaps hers wasn't so bad after all.'

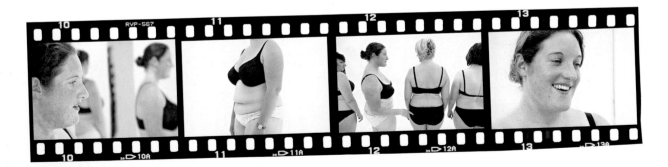

'I'm 26 years old. I'm nice. I'm normal. I just want to feel sexy and to have a boyfriend.'

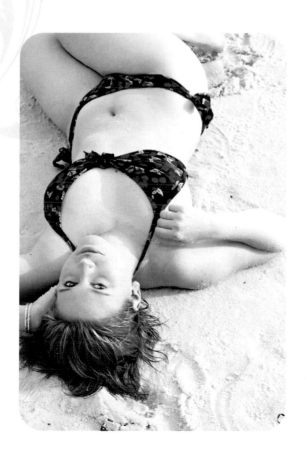

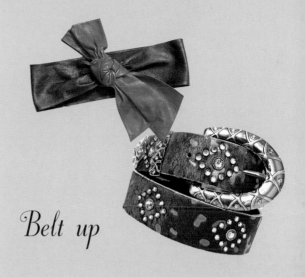

Belt up

Focusing on your waist is a great way of creating some curves, no matter what size you are. But it's important to choose the right belt for your shape. Here's how:

- Hourglass: a waist-cinching belt brings the eye to the smallest part of you – your waist.
- Apple: tops with belted embroidery and detail that sits under your breasts will elongate your waist and even make your legs look longer.
- Pear: you're best off avoiding belts, although very thin ones looped through your trousers or jeans are okay. Otherwise, like the apple, opt for empire-line tops to elongate those pins.
- Pencil: avoid wide and stiff belts and choose softer materials, such as ribbons, or belted cardigans.

THE POSTER TEST

Ally's body-loathing had gone on for so long that this time we needed something more radical than a simple makeover. We needed to shock her into seeing just how other people saw her: sexy, curvy and beautiful.

Ally was bowled over by the comments. 'It felt so strange to hear those compliments, and know that we didn't pay any of them to say those things!'

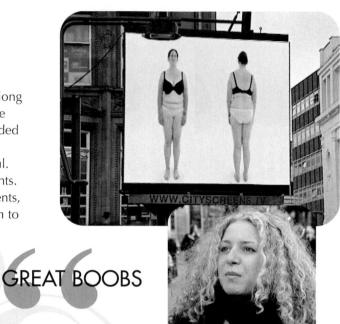

GREAT BOOBS

BIG BOOBS
REALLY SEXY

GREAT LEGS – THERE'S NO CELLULITE

THE MAKEOVER

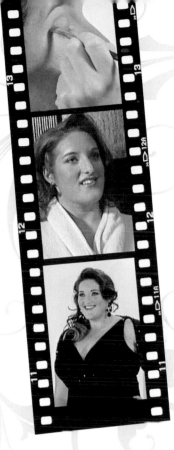

Ally had taken many comments to heart and begun to pay more attention to herself and her appearance. In just six weeks she'd lost two and a half stone and was spending more time getting ready when she went out. Even her friends had noticed the difference in her attitude. But she still lacked confidence when it came to men and dressing to impress.

'My rule when it came to buying clothes that as long as it was comfortable, then it was doing its job,' she said. For Ally it was never a question of whether an outfit suited her or made her look more attractive. The more flesh was covered, the more suitable it was.

We showed Ally that dressing to flatter your figure is all about hiding the lumps and bumps you don't want others to see, and highlighting the parts of yourself that are alluring and attractive. Ally's collarbone was beautiful, and highlighting it was a great way to shift attention away from her wider hips and bottom. Wide, sexy shoulders that taper down to a small, womanly waist are a sure-fire way to grab some attention. Off the shoulder or V-necked tops were perfect for her – they gave her instant shape and sex appeal and meant she no longer looked like the square shape she'd been dressing as. Tops that finished or tapered in at the waistline also helped to create some serious curves. In short, our job was to make an hourglass out of a pear.

ALLY'S PERFECT OUTFIT

We showed Ally that skinny jeans aren't just for skinny girls. Well-cut denim can create a stylish, sexy silhouette. We added some high heels and a wide belt that pulled in her waist even further and emphasized her beautiful boobs and lovely hips and bum. With a seasonal coat and party handbag Ally was ready to party. And it worked – her new-found confidence in herself and her appearance meant that she quickly bagged herself a boyfriend!

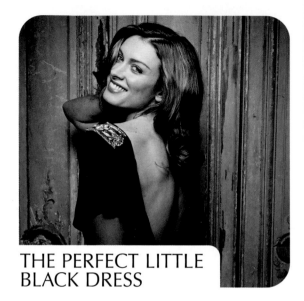

THE PERFECT LITTLE BLACK DRESS

The little black number is a party staple, but you need to find out what suits you:

Wide hips
A fitted, figure-hugging top will hit all the right notes. Team with a wrap or sheer blouse if you want to hide your arms.

Small shoulders
V-neck dresses will create curves and soften your bony shoulders.

Lack of waist
Party dresses with a wide sash will draw the eye to the waist. Ruched waists are another great option.

Heavy thighs
Detailed necklines will focus the attention away from your boxy shape.

MAKE-UP HINTS AND TIPS FOR PARTY GIRLS

If you're heading out for a night of fun, then make sure that your make-up lasts as long as you do. Follow the guidelines below for the best results:

- It's important to create a good base, so use a good moisturizer suitable for your skin, and apply a primer on top. This helps to reduce oily T-zones, and keep your foundation in place.

- Your night-time foundation shouldn't feel like you are putting on a mask. Remember, less is more. Just cover up any blemishes or red areas and let your natural beauty shine through.

- Make up your eyes or lips with this season's colours – never both.

- Apply your heated eyelash curlers to open those peepers, and then apply mascara. Once you've got your eyes defined, you'll have a better idea of how much eyeshadow, liner and contouring you need.

- If you've gone all out on the eyeshadow, then a touch of tinted lipgloss is all you need for your perfect pout.

- Don't forget your rouge – a lighter colour above your cheekbones will give you an instant lift.

- Keep your face powder on standby. This is your secret weapon to keeping party-fresh all night long. So put it in your handbag. Now.

Salon Style

FACIAL WAXING

It's not just the boys who get stubble trouble. If you've got some facial hair, then don't ignore it. There are ways and means! If hair has suddenly appeared on your lip, chin or jawline, then it may be due to hormonal changes in your body, so visit your GP to check. But if you've always had a little fur, then there's nothing to be ashamed of. Just learn how to keep it under control and out of sight. Whatever you do, don't pluck unwanted facial hair (other than on your eyebrows), as this will just encourage growth. Instead, visit a beauty salon for guidance and choose between the following:

Waxing

One of the most popular solutions.

Ideal for removing hair on the upper lip and fine hair on the side of the face.

Avoid waxing your chin area. If you have darker skin, then waxing can cause discolouration and irritation.

Lasts for two to six weeks.

Electrolysis

Uses low-level electricity to kill the hair follicles. Can be time consuming and costly.

Ideal for fine, blonde hair and for removing hair on the upper lip and chin.

Avoid if you're looking for a budget solution. Ensure you always go to a reputable salon.

Lasts for up to two months – or longer after a few sessions.

Laser

New, but a goodie. Uses a laser to eliminate hair.

Ideal for those with fair skin and dark hair.

Avoid if you're fair-haired – laser hair removal may not be as effective.

Effectiveness 50 to 70% reduction after three treatments, performed six weeks apart.

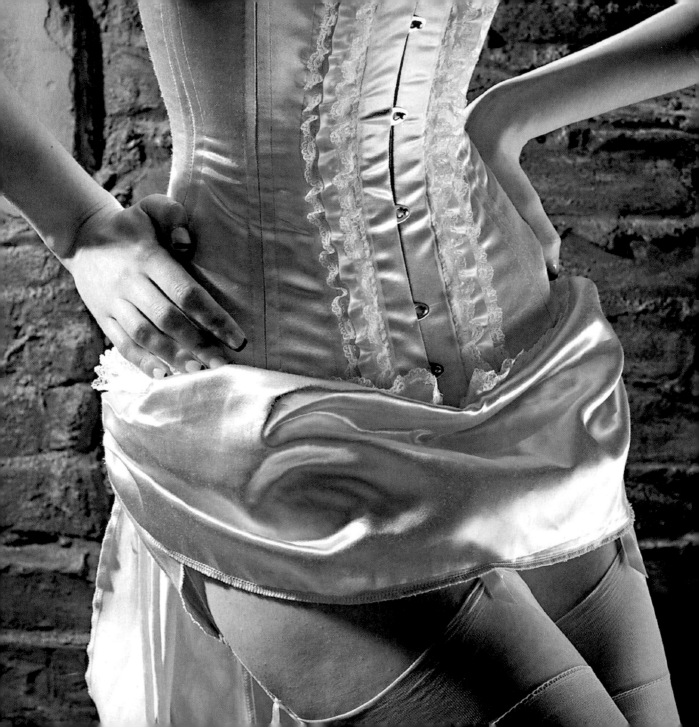

SCULPTING WITHOUT SURGERY

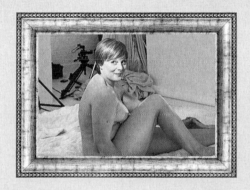

Roberta Fox Braddock, 49, lived in South Wales, and worked at a steel plant. She'd been married to Jonathan for 23 years but disliked her body so much that it got in the way of their sex life. Roberta needed to learn how to dress her body to wow the pants off her husband. She hated her bum and dressed in big, baggy clothes, which only made her derriere look bigger.

And her bitterness over her bottom was even affecting her social life. Instead of going out on romantic dates with her husband, Roberta hid inside and kept her rear out of view. What Roberta wanted most of all – even more than a smaller bum – was to become invisible.

We had our work cut out. We needed to show Roberta that it was ok to dress in a way that would make people sit up and notice how beautiful she was. The last time Roberta had worn a dress was seven years ago. Our job was to put some wow back into her wardrobe and dress with confidence and – ultimately – to feel confident butt naked.

IN THE MIRROR

Roberta, like seven out of 10 women in the UK, hates her bum. To help her understand how distorted her body image was, we forced her to look at herself properly in the mirror, without clothes. At first it was difficult to persuade her to get naked. 'All I see is wobble,' she said. 'Everything is wobbly. My bottom is two great big pads of fat and it's sort of broad and it sticks out. It's just too big.' Even though Roberta's hourglass body shape does mean she's widest at the bottom and hips, she actually doesn't have a wide bottom per se. All her bum needed was a lift and then a bit of shape – without going under the knife.

BODY PERCEPTION

Roberta had no true idea of what her body looked liked. She'd blown her posterior problems all out of proportion. In fact, she had a very average-sized 44-inch bum, and a sexy, shapely one at that. In our line-up of gorgeous girls, she placed herself near the bigger end of the bottoms – and gave herself an extra four inches on her rear. By not being realistic about her bottom, Roberta was imagining that she was almost two dress sizes bigger than she really was. And yet half the passers-by we surveyed said that Roberta's best asset was her arse!

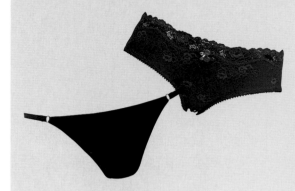

Naughty knickers

Bums come in all shapes and sizes, so dress yours in the most flattering, sexiest style.

- Thongs: any bottom can wear a g-string, as long as it's firm. But if you can't bear the thought of a dental flossing, but still need an invisible panty line under your clothes, then knickers with a flat lace trim are a great alternative.

- Boy shorts: ideal for wearing with low-rise trousers. But steer clear if you've got thunder thighs, as they'll just cut you off at your widest point.

- French knickers: these are best left in the bedroom, as they're uber sexy. Great for hiding a multitude of sins though!

THE MAKEOVER

Roberta's intense dislike of her own body shape meant that she'd ignored all femininity. Yet by dressing Roberta in the correct underwear, we gave her a boob lift, leg and tummy liposuction and a couple of bum implants! We knew that her pear shape would look fabulous in a full-length frock. Once we'd got evening glamour sorted, daywear was a doddle. A shift dress with a light chiffon top half worked well. A skirt with hidden pleats was another success. The right outfit for the office was particularly important for Roberta. She was thrilled with a very structured, bright red jacket and slimming black trousers that immediately said 'confidence' and 'control'.

FABULOUS FROCKS

If, like Roberta, you need a bit of help in the bum area, a bias-cut, backless dress that kicks

'I hated being miserable all the time, because it affected all the people I love the most.'

out at the hem will give you a better shape, and balance out your bum. Here are a few frock tips (see p.29 for more):

- If you're tall and slender small floral prints will look great on you. If you have a fuller figure, then larger prints will be more slimming.

- Lace fabric is perfect for transforming boyish or athletic shapes into sexy, feminine silhouettes.

- If you have a few wobbly bits, then chiffon material will float over them.

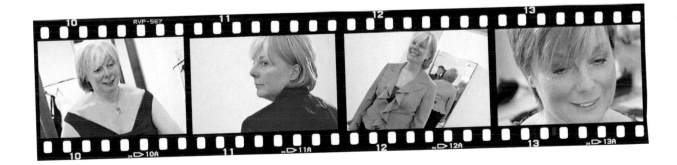

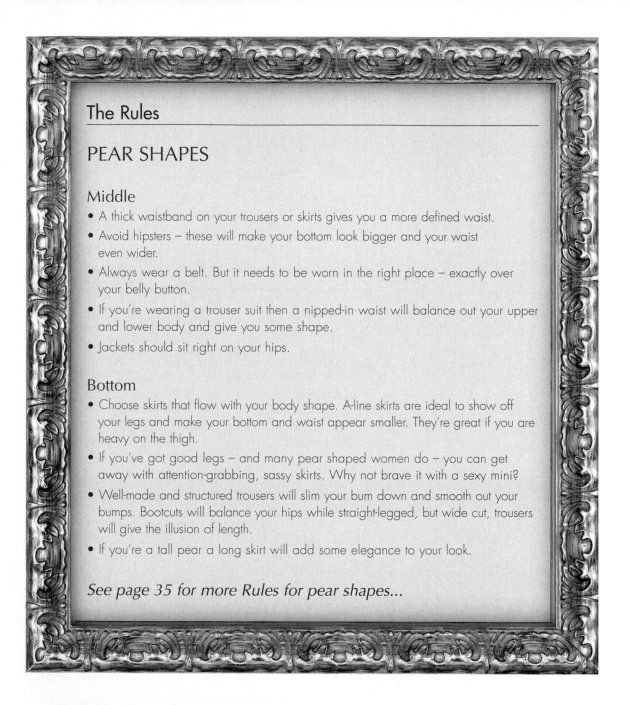

The Rules

PEAR SHAPES

Middle

- A thick waistband on your trousers or skirts gives you a more defined waist.
- Avoid hipsters – these will make your bottom look bigger and your waist even wider.
- Always wear a belt. But it needs to be worn in the right place – exactly over your belly button.
- If you're wearing a trouser suit then a nipped-in waist will balance out your upper and lower body and give you some shape.
- Jackets should sit right on your hips.

Bottom

- Choose skirts that flow with your body shape. A-line skirts are ideal to show off your legs and make your bottom and waist appear smaller. They're great if you are heavy on the thigh.
- If you've got good legs – and many pear shaped women do – you can get away with attention-grabbing, sassy skirts. Why not brave it with a sexy mini?
- Well-made and structured trousers will slim your bum down and smooth out your bumps. Bootcuts will balance your hips while straight-legged, but wide cut, trousers will give the illusion of length.
- If you're a tall pear a long skirt will add some elegance to your look.

See page 35 for more Rules for pear shapes...

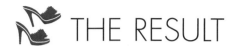

THE RESULT

We showed Roberta how well-cut, structured clothes would allow her to dress stylishly and simply during the day in tailored suits and dresses, and to add a few accessories, such as glittery boleros, clutch bags and dancing shoes, in the evening to make the switch from office girl to party-maker. A shorter, layered haircut accentuated her high cheekbones and made her neck look more slender and elegant. The pièce de résistance was a day of treatments: body wrap, pedicure and spray tan. A bit of pampering goes a long way when it comes to boosting your confidence.

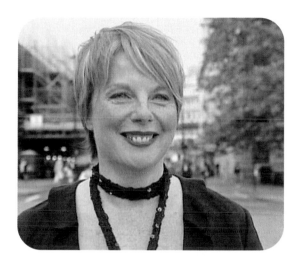

Salon Style

HOW TO LOOK AFTER A PEAR-SHAPE BUM

Never yo yo diet if you are a pear shape. This just leads to weight gain on your bottom, while your top will remain slender. And dieting leads to sagging and dimpling of the skin, which will make you dislike your bottom even more.

If your skin is dry, then add some softness by applying body moisturizer within three minutes of getting out of the shower. This will ensure your skin seals in the benefits of the cream or oil and looks and feels silky smooth.

Walking, running or anything that keeps toning those butt muscles are an everyday beauty must.

Eat lots of oily fish: not only will you be brainier, but your bottom will be better for it, as its essential fatty acids help your skin appear and feel smoother, so no more orange peel bottoms!

Trousers

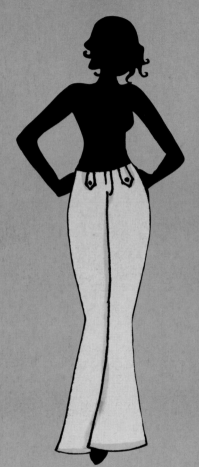

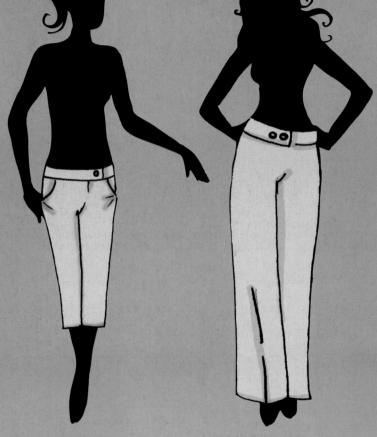

FLARED
FEATURES: kick out from the knee
GOOD FOR: pear, hourglass
BAD FOR: apple

CROPPED
FEATURES: end mid-calf
GOOD FOR: pencil
BAD FOR: pear, hourglass, apple

WIDE, STRAIGHT-LEGGED
FEATURES: skim hips and fall to the floor
GOOD FOR: all shapes
BAD FOR: none

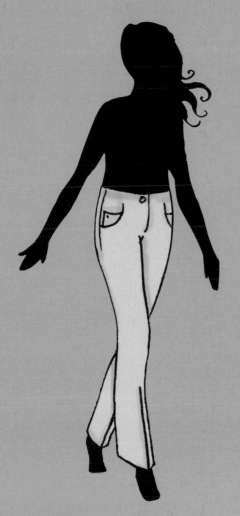

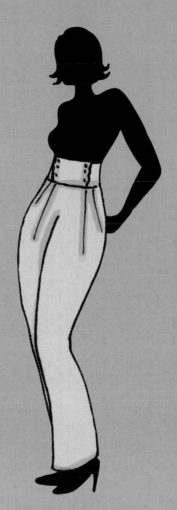

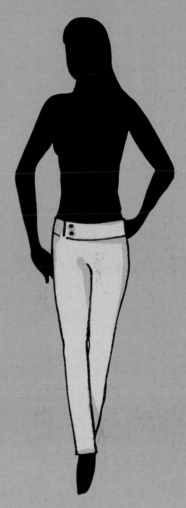

BOOT CUT

FEATURES: kick out slightly below the knee
GOOD FOR: pear, hourglass, apple
BAD FOR: pencil

HIGH-WAISTED

FEATURES: pull tummies in
GOOD FOR: pear, hourglass, apple
BAD FOR: some pencils

PENCIL

FEATURES: tight-fitting
GOOD FOR: pencil
BAD FOR: pear, hourglass, apple

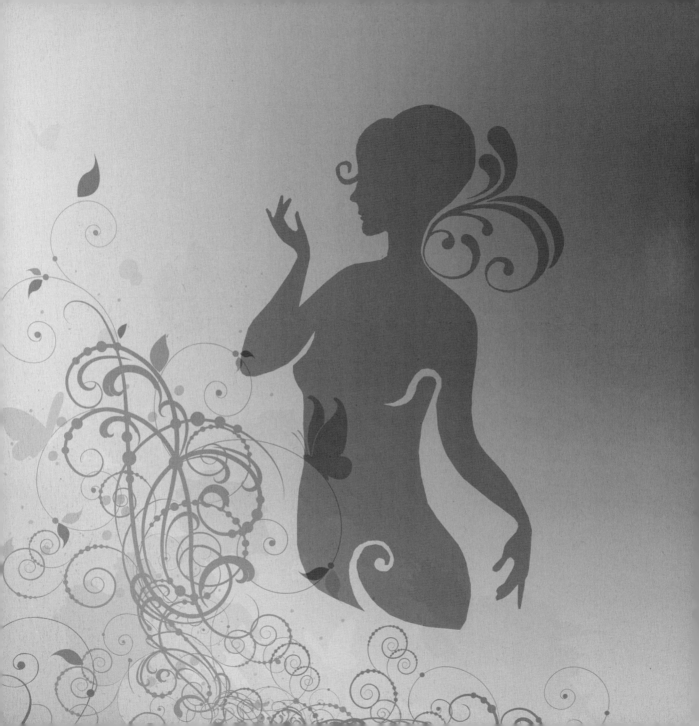

Chapter 5

ALL-OVER BODY BLUES

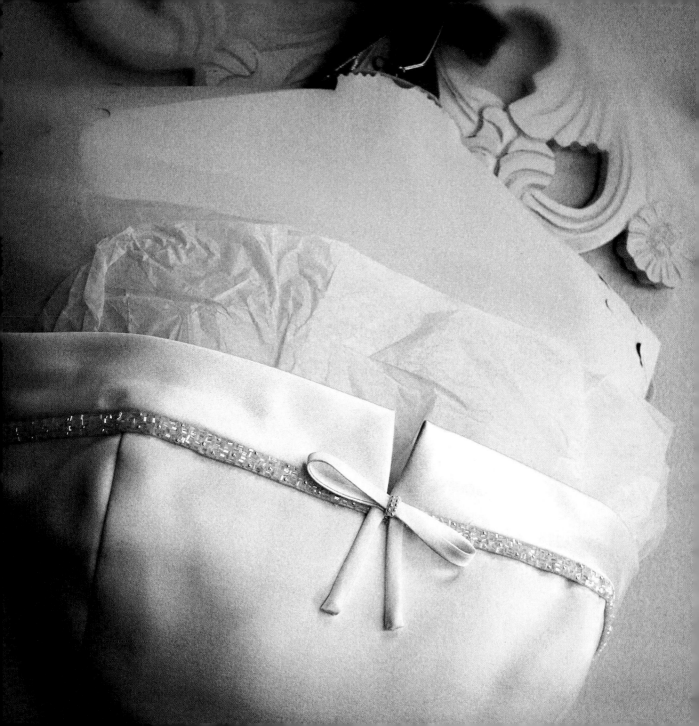

PETITE ALL OVER

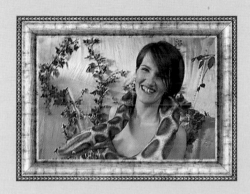

Jenny Stockton, 26, was a mother of two children from Cheshire who was in crisis; she didn't even have her own distinct wardrobe. Instead, she wore her boyfriend Simon's clothes, even though her tiny but perfectly formed frame got completely lost under his voluminous outfits and baggy fleeces. Both Jenny and her partner Simon lived in oversized sweaters and tracksuit pants that did nothing for their bodies or their floundering love life.

Jenny was a petite size 8 – the sort of size most women dream of being. She didn't own a full-length mirror so had no idea what she looked like. In fact, she wouldn't even look at her face, let alone her whole body. Her reflection was something to be avoided at all costs.

Partner Simon was tall and thin with a body that was made for the catwalk, but it was difficult to see his sporty frame under his oversized sweaters. In terms of their outfits, the couple were completely indistinguishable from each other. We made it our mission to banish their joint wardrobe and get them both looking good together, dressed and naked.

WHAT SHE SAW

Jenny hadn't looked in a mirror for 10 years and hadn't worn a bra for eight years. 'There's not much point to me,' she said. 'I'm a mum, and there's a point to that, but not much point to me. I don't wear a bra because my boobs are small and saggy and there's nothing to put into the cups. I don't even know what my bra size is.' Jenny didn't think that she deserved to wear a bra and to look and feel womanly. Her oversized clothes meant that nobody else got to see her fabulous figure, and the stupid thing was, Jenny admitted to not even liking her comfort clothes. Simon thought she was gorgeous though. 'I love her body, it's absolutely beautiful, as simple as that,' he said. It would be a lot of effort to persuade Jenny to think the same way. It was clearly essential to get her boob issue sorted first.

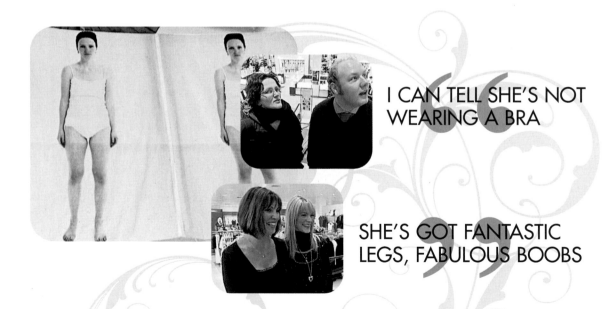

I CAN TELL SHE'S NOT WEARING A BRA

SHE'S GOT FANTASTIC LEGS, FABULOUS BOOBS

SHE'S IN GOOD PROPORTION WITH A LOVELY SLIM FIGURE

BODY PERCEPTION

We lined up five small-breasted women, all of whom were wearing A-cups but in varying styles and shapes. This was to show Jenny that a different cut could really make a different to the appearance of your cleavage. In the UK 47% of women say they are unhappy with their breasts. But many of these women could do a lot by choosing a bra style that really enhances their assets (see box, right).

Finally, Jenny uttered the words we had been longing to hear: 'Time to go and buy a bra.' We chose a wonderful padded push-up bra and Jenny was transformed from flat chested to curvy beauty. Simon was delighted. 'I think it's fabulous that Jenny is finally wearing a bra,' he said. 'She looks great and so sexy.

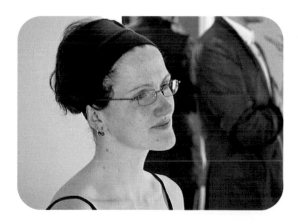

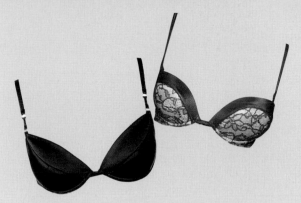

Bras for small boobs

Small-breasted women should never go without a bra. The right size bra will not only support your breasts, but various shapes and styles can add curves and even give you a cleavage. Here's how:

- Underwired bras will help to lift your boobs if they've dropped a little.
- Padding can create more curves than you've ever seen before!
- Chicken fillets are great for inserting into your bra. These push your boobs up and together and give some alluring cleavage.
- Balcony bras have cushioning to give even the smallest breasts lift and add the illusion of a cup size. Balcony bras look gorgeously glamorous under rounded low-cut tops and sculpt and enhance small chests really well.
- Remember the bottom half too. If you've got no bum, then padded knickers give you some sexy bottom curves to match the ones up top.

THE MAKEOVER

Jenny's striking red hair and fantastic figure meant we could be bold with colours, shapes and patterns. Skinny jeans were made for Jenny's long, slender legs. We chose to team them with black, patent heels – the hem sat at Jenny's ankle for an up-to-the-minute way to wear skinnies. If your legs are on the shorter side, then let the jean or pant hem hang over your heels.

Jenny and Simon had a unique, slightly offbeat style, which we didn't want to stifle. So we matched her faded denims with a trendy red tartan jacket. The jacket cinched in her tiny waist and kicked out enough to accentuate her hips. A 60s sex siren was born.

As for Simon, out went the big baggy clothes and in came a sharp Prince of Wales suit teamed with purple silk shirt and a smooth pork pie hat. They made a seriously handsome pair.

To help boost Jenny's girly wardrobe, we introduced a bright red dress teamed with an acid blue belt to cinch in her waist. If you're small boned, then dresses are your new best friend as they can help to create curves as well as hide any bumps.

A make-up lesson taught Jenny how to make the most of her delicate facial features and to feel like the incredibly pretty girl she was. If you feel uncomfortable wearing too much make-up, then less really is more. A well-shaped pair of eyebrows, curled eyelashes with mascara and some shine-eliminating powder with tinted lipgloss is all you need. Jenny loved her new 'natural' look and began to feel more and more womanly. A professional blowdry and Jenny was virtually unrecognizable from the shy and retiring woman we'd met a few weeks earlier.

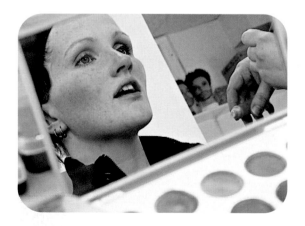

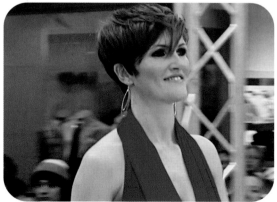

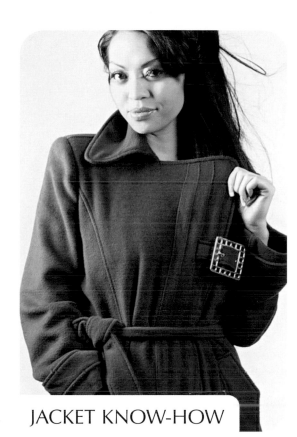

JACKET KNOW-HOW

If it's cold out you don't need to hide under unflattering baggy jumpers. The right style of jacket for your shape can give you curves and a sexy silhouette, and it's a great way to finish off your look.

Apple

This shape does tend to have trouble with jackets, but there are some successful options. An A-line, swing jacket is perfect to skim lumps and bumps. Opt for softer lines, not severe military style cuts, and look for medium-weight fabrics, otherwise you're adding extra unnecessary inches.

Pear

Blazers are great, as the structure will give you hourglass-like curves. Your jacket should sit on the hip, any longer and your hips will look too wide. Lighter colours will draw the eye upwards and teamed with dark trousers will help balance out your proportions.

Hourglass

Single-breasted jackets that do up right under your ribs will draw attention to your tiny waist. Avoid double-breasted cuts, as these can make you look top heavy. Lapels shouldn't be too wide.

Flat chested

Layering is your best friend. A couple of layers of close-fitting streamlined tops and a lightweight tailored jacket is ideal. Add a belt for some waistline detail or pockets, which give you sexy curves. Double-breasted jackets will give the illusion of larger breasts. Avoid anything baggy, as it will overwhelm your frame.

Top heavy

Vertical striped jackets will elongate your shape. Jackets with a small print are particularly good for you.

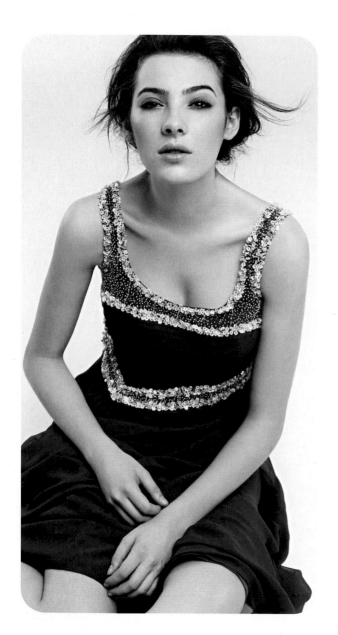

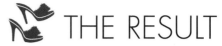 # THE RESULT

Jenny and Simon made over their wardrobe, their look and their lives in just six weeks. By dressing for their body shape, rather than for what was easiest to grab from their joint wardrobe, they transformed their confidence levels and did great things for their relationship. 'I like the way I look, I think I look nice now. I feel so confident and sexy and beautiful. I never thought I would feel like this,' Jenny said. 'Jenny managed to overcome quite a lot of

'I like the way I look, I think I look nice now. I feel so confident and sexy and beautiful.'

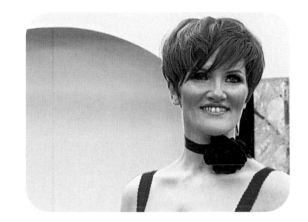

demons and really shone,' said Simon. 'I think we both look fab now!'

The pair celebrated their new look with a daring display in the window of an Oxford Street store – they posed naked as Adam and Eve, complete with serpents! They looked so fantastic tempting passers-by with their buff and beautiful bodies.

Salon Style

MALE BEAUTY

The male beauty market has seen an explosion in recent years. Across the globe men now spend an extraordinary £800m a year on personal grooming products, with skincare sales making up a significant proportion of this. Here's how to help the man in your life make the most of his skin:

If he shaves daily he needs to replace lost moisture with a lightweight moisturizer that is right for his skin type.

He should avoid moisturizing the chin and nose. This can lead to ingrown hairs and blackheads.

Urge him to invest in an eye cream, or at least use his moisturizer around the eye area.

A cleanser for his skin is also great – it doesn't have to be anything fancy. Cold cream will do the job.

Make sure he never forgets sunscreen. It will keep wrinkles at bay and protect the skin from sun damage.

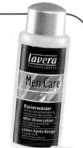

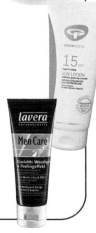

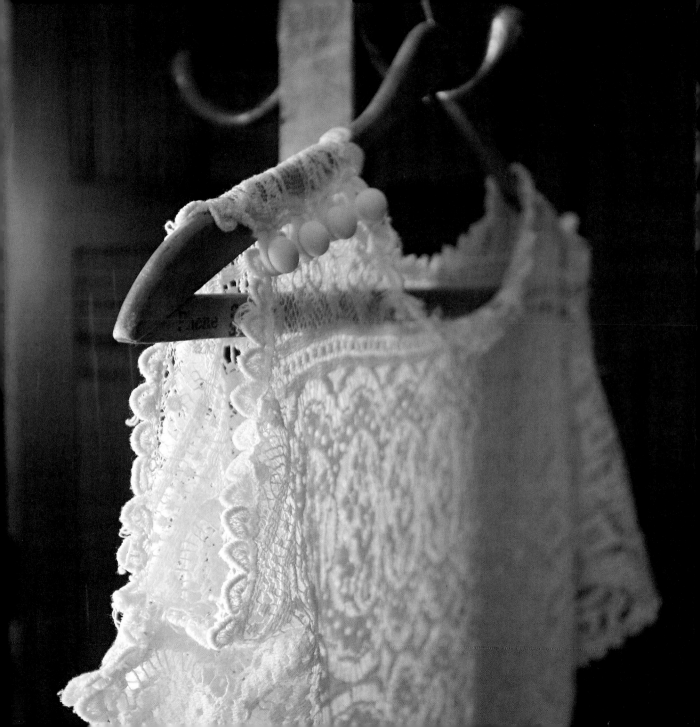

HAND-ME-DOWN HIPPY

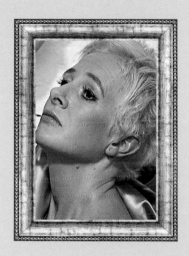

Lisa Mayall, 36, a self-confessed hippy from Newbury in Berkshire, had let herself go in more ways than one. A single mum of three children, Lisa certainly had little time for herself, and things like pampering or shopping for clothes just didn't come into the equation. Lisa existed in shapeless hand-me-downs that did nothing to flatter her gorgeous figure. It had been so long though since anybody, even Lisa, had seen her naked, that she had forgotten just how shapely and sexy she was.

Lisa's body image problems, or rather her body blindness, didn't stop at her wardrobe. She also paid very little attention to her hair: on her head, and on the rest of her body. Having visited the hairdresser just once in the last three years, her topknot was in danger of turning into a topiary. Her bikini line needed some attention too!

We embarked upon a regime of serious body maintenance – not just to help Lisa look better naked but to make her comfortable enough to reveal all in front of somebody special.

◯ WHAT SHE SAW

Lisa knew that her fear of facing her naked image was seriously holding her back and was part of the reason she that her life was in such a rut. She was at least sufficiently self-aware to realise that her body confidence was a problem for her, and stopped her from going out and meeting people.

When it came to confronting the glass, Lisa became simply sick with nerves. 'Things sag – gravity has caught up with me,' she said. 'I never look at myself.' Her prized possession seemed to be some curtains that her mum made her – because she could hide the mirror behind them. In fact, the last time anybody had seen Lisa naked was more than three years earlier. Ultimately, she feared being alone for the rest of her life.

Once she did sneak a peak, however, she was astounded by how hairy she was! 'I have hairy armpits, hairy legs. I look more hairy than I thought I would,' she confessed.

But there was a different side to the story. Undressed, Lisa revealed a gorgeous size 10 figure that could really carry off something

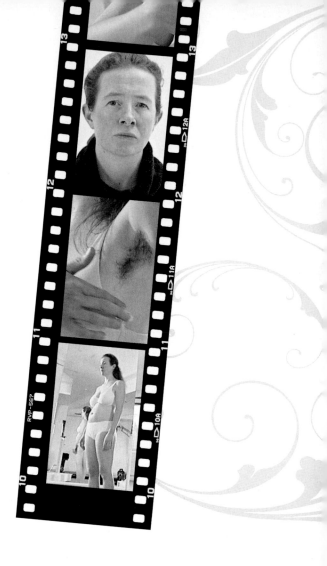

'*I doubt that many people really know what I look like underneath my baggy clothes.*'

special. If she didn't want to spend any more nights in alone, then it was time she did something about her hair issue and unleashed her fantastic body on the world.

Lisa's biggest hang-up was her tummy. At a teensy weensy 30 inches, Lisa's waist was four inches smaller than the national average. Despite having such a tiny tum, Lisa believed she was six inches larger and so had been wearing size 14 clothes for years and dressing two sizes larger. She genuinely believed that this was what she looked like.

The fact was, Lisa was a complete clothes horse – she had the sort of body that could look good in anything! Except she didn't know it.

THE POSTER TEST

The first step to convincing Lisa that she had an enviable figure was to hit the streets of Newbury. First, we asked people what they thought of her figure underneath one of her classic shapeless jumpers. The response was, of course, that they didn't think anything – they couldn't see her. But when we revealed all, and projected a 50-foot tall poster of Lisa's body on the streets of her home town, we got an unanimous response. Lisa was luscious!

It was essential that Lisa begin to see what other people saw when they looked at her body: a fabulous, womanly shape with beautiful features. Her wardrobe makeover would be key.

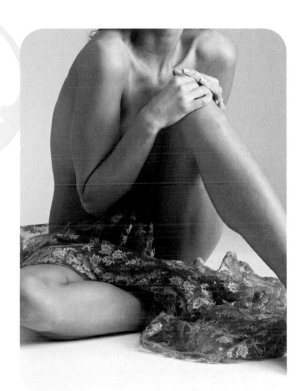

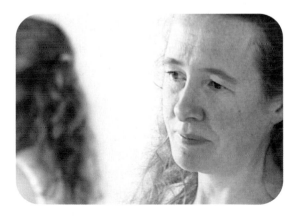

THE MAKEOVER

As a small size 10, Lisa could wear almost any style. We began our new wardrobe search in the denim department to show Lisa that jeans can look sexy and stylish. A loose, flared jean in washed denim gave her a fabulous base to add some sexy summer tops. We teamed these with a soft tailored jacket and a fashionable belt.

Lisa's body shape was so adaptable that skinny jeans looked great too. We added knee-high stiletto boots, a gathered smock top and – the final touch – a cropped leather jacket to draw attention to her waspish waist and bring her look bang up-to-date.

For a more romantic look, we teamed the same skinny jeans with a demure black vest and cardigan. Matched with bright yellow heels and belt, Lisa at last looked ready to go on a date.

The anti-ageing market is worth £650 million and continues to grow.

But we still had to address Lisa's hair issue! We waxed her armpits, bikini line and legs, something that was totally alien to her. It was a revelation! 'I love it, this is the way I want to look,' she said.

With two weeks to go before her catwalk appearance, she had taken down the curtain in front of her mirror, joined a Pilates class and returned her charity shop cast-offs.

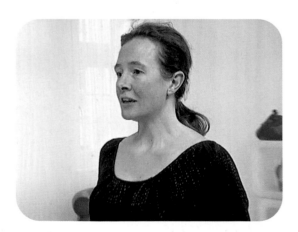
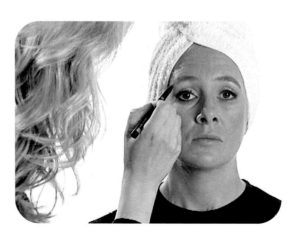

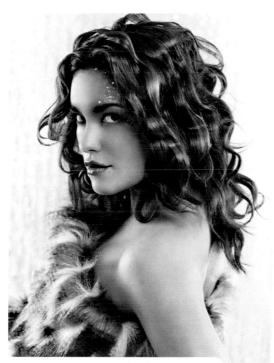

HAIRSTYLES FOR BODY SHAPES

The right hairstyle can work just like a well-structured jacket, making you look thinner, younger and more fashionable. But which hair cut would suit your body shape? Here's our handy guide:

Petite
Go for a slightly wavy, shoulder-length cut. Avoid anything too childlike, such as ponytails or fancy hair accessories. A fringe may make you look even shorter, so avoid.

Larger figures
Go for a medium-length style with long layers around the face. Don't go too short, as this can make your face look fuller. Wispy fringes can soften your features and draw attention to your eyes.

Pencil
Big hair with big curls is ideal. So heat up those rollers and think big!

Pear
Balance out your wider hips with choppy layers that add volume. Shoulder-length styles are best.

Apple
Avoid anything too pixieish or wispy, as these styles will make your head look too small. Longer styles will draw the eye downwards and make your shoulders look less broad.

Hourglass
Anything goes for this shape, so work with your hairdresser to find a look that suits your face shape and be prepared to experiment.

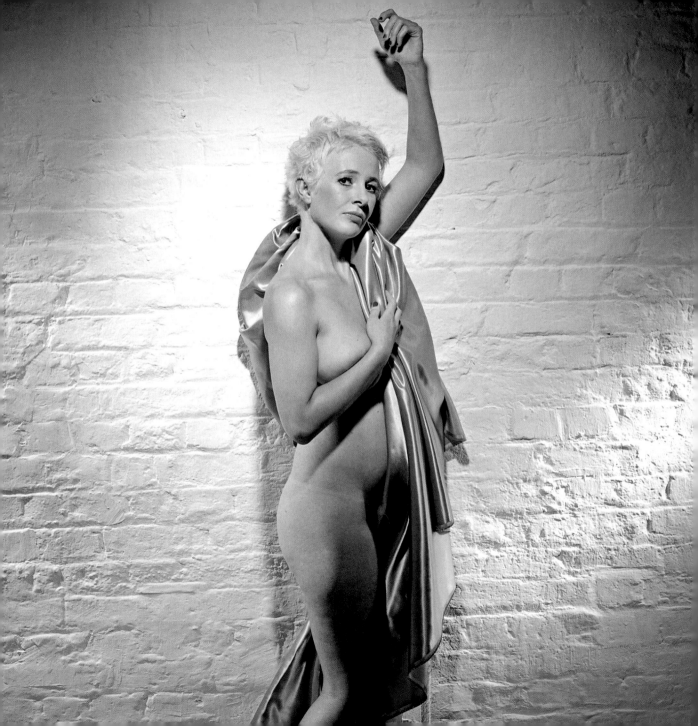

THE RESULT

Lisa's stylish new look flaunted the latest fashions perfectly and she looked fab in her beautiful black, sexy underwear. To help Lisa look and feel fabulous even when naked, we chopped off her reliable ponytail and hit the bottle instead. Bleached blonde hair would ensure that she would turn heads wherever she went. With a top-to-toe wax and some flattering underwear there was no sign of the hairy hippy. 'This is the me that has been hiding for far too long,' she said. 'I'm confident, much happier. I like looking at my tummy now.' And after a successful naked photo shoot, Lisa had just one more challenge facing her: to strut her stuff on the catwalk.

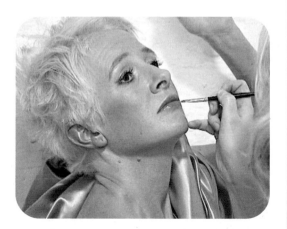

BIKINI-LINE KNOW-HOW

The best way to remove unwanted hair from the bikini line is by waxing or sugaring. These gives the smoothest results and you'll be less likely to get ingrown hairs, red bumps or irritation. Best of all, the results last for at least four weeks – so your bikini line will see you through your holiday and more. Although it is possible to do your own, for the best results visit a beautician. Remember, don't get your bikini line waxed just before your period.

In the UK 83% of women trim their bikini lines. But only 14% go for the full Brazilian. So which bikini line would suit your shape?

Apple: Brazilian (or 'landing-strip')
The vertical line draws the eye to the centre of the body, rather than to its width.

Hourglass: clean-shaven
The eye is not distracted with any bikini-line hair: make the most of those curves!

Pear: V-shape
This will balance out the lower body and de-emphasize the hips.

Pencil: natural
This will add some softness to your shape. But you still have to maintain it!

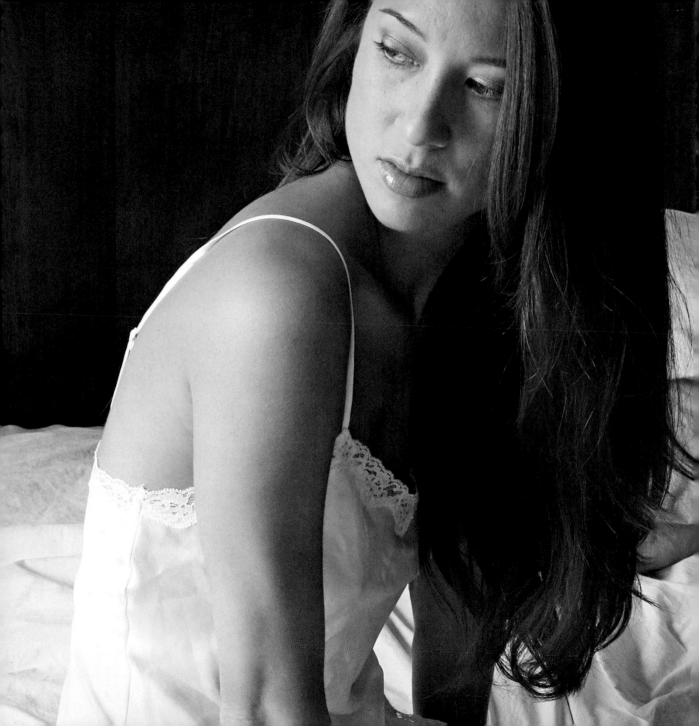

HEIGHT HANG-UPS

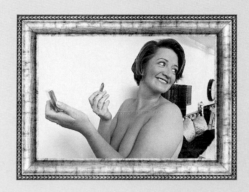

Rachel Richardson, 39, was a theatre nurse who had run out of patience. The ultimate body hater, she saw herself more as a bloke in drag than the buxom beauty she really was. At 5 feet 10 inches tall Rachel felt that she towered over everybody else, and that her size 14 figure made her stick out like a sore thumb. Her height and her dress size made her believe that she was stocky and manly, so she hid her figure under shapeless t-shirts, jumpers and baggy jeans, which did nothing for her figure. At work, Rachel chose the biggest and baggiest scrubs to hide her curves, believing that this would make her appear shorter and smaller.

Rachel's perception of herself as unfeminine and unsexy coincided with the approach of the big four-o. She desperately wanted to be at peace with her body but constantly put herself down to her family and friends. Rachel rarely went out with partner Adrian, sometimes refusing to leave the house because she thought she looked so dreadful. She had refused Adrian's offers of marriage for fear of what she would look like on the big day.

◎ IN THE MIRROR

Most women hanker after more height. In fact, in the UK a massive 87.5% of women want to be taller. Yet Rachel just wanted to shrink herself down. Her trip to the mirror room was emotional and teary. 'I'm just too big, too boring,' she said. 'I'd much rather be normal. I just want to be a normal size.' It was Rachel's dream to wear high heels, but as they made her more than six feet tall she wore flat, uninspiring footwear instead. Somebody had once compared her to a man and it seemed she had never recovered from that. She believed that

In the UK, a massive 87.5% of women want to be taller.

everyone saw her as big, bulky and butch. Until she accepted herself, height and all, and learnt to have a happy relationship with herself, she would never be able to have one with others.

BODY PERCEPTION

A line-up of lean lovelies outfitted in hospital scrubs showed Rachel just how large and unappealing she looked in her daily uniform. Yet undressed, each and every one of those women had a sexy, shapely figure. What Rachel didn't realize was that they were also all a size 14 like her. It was a revelation to Rachel that size 14 could mean sexy, not oversized. It started to dawn on her that she really wasn't such a freak.

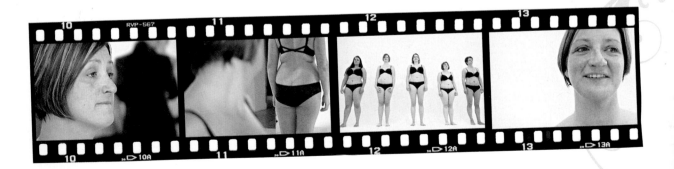

THE MAKEOVER

Our first step was to show Rachel how it was possible for someone of her shape to dress in a womanly and feminine style. Her closet was full of ill-fitting clothes, with a strange mixture of items that were either too small or too baggy, and virtually nothing that actually fit her hourglass figure! Every day Rachel chose to ignore her body shape for what it was and made herself even more depressed in the process.

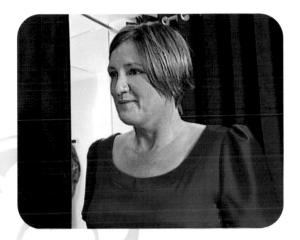

We had to show Rachel that her hourglass was stunning and that her height, far from taking away from this, made her silhouette even more striking. We went for a pair of skinny jeans and matched these with a figure-hugging ¾-length top, which helped to balance her endless legs by elongating her torso. The thigh-skimming top also sat neatly on her bottom, which hid it from view, but suggested that it was pert and perfect. Even though Rachel was self-conscious about her height, we taught her that tall meant beautiful, not boyish. We added heels, which is the right thing to do even if you are tall, otherwise your outfit will look unfinished. Rachel was impressed, even though she had an unusual way of expressing it: 'It feels different to look in the mirror and not want to vomit. It takes a bit of getting used to,' she said. Partner Adrian was blown away. 'I think she looks beautiful, gorgeous,' he said.

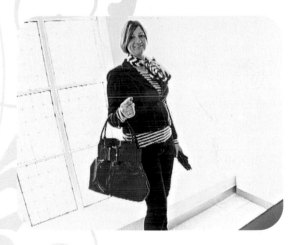

Another really successful outfit for Rachel was an attention-grabbing purple jewelled dress and slimming black opaque tights (with secret support from her magic knickers of course!). She had categorically avoided nights out, so embarrassed was she by her body, but the knockout purple number was a big step on the way to feeling comfortable with her head-turning shape. She hit the town and, for the first time, loved the attention she got.

In the past Rachel had done all she could to avoid people looking at her: at just shy of 40 she felt old, tired and knackered looking. After a stint in hair and make-up, she was ready to adorn her very own window display on London's Oxford Street. Although she was terrified of being seen naked sitting down, we showed her how she could stand in a sexy, alluring way. 'This has done so much for my confidence,' said a delighted Rachel.

'I would never have dreamt of getting naked in front of a bunch of strangers a few weeks ago. I've definitely changed!'

The Rules

TALL AND LONG SHAPES

- If you're lucky enough to be a leggy lovely, don't spoil it by stooping! Embrace your height and hold your head up high.

- It's a myth that heels are not for you. They will make you stand up straight and stop you stooping, so strap on those skyscrapers.

- Wear detailed tops to draw attention upwards.

- If you are a tall pear shape, horizontal stripes on top are very good at balancing out your figure.

- Avoid vertical stripes; they will just make you look longer.

- Wear black or dark-coloured bottoms with a lighter top if you're self-conscious about the size of your butt.

- Go for wide-cut tops that show off your shapely shoulders and make your neck appear slim.

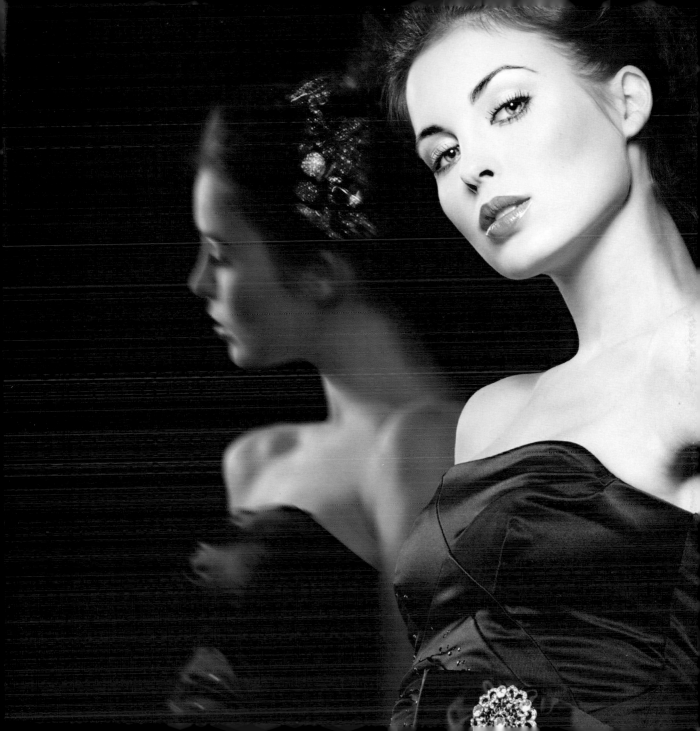

THE RESULT

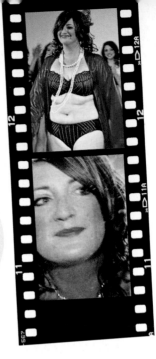

As the final test of Rachel's newfound confidence, we unleashed her on the catwalk to shake her booty. To give her some extra femininity and great movement we added some hair extensions. Good extensions shouldn't be noticeable, so shop around for a trustworthy hairdresser who can advise you on what works for your shape, style and personality. With a floor-length stunning red dress and some serious bling, Rachel's transformation was complete. She also flaunted her figure in gorgeous underwear – with her held high and shoulders pulled back, she looked like a supermodel.

Rachel's confidence was so sky high that she capped it all by proposing to Adrian on the catwalk!

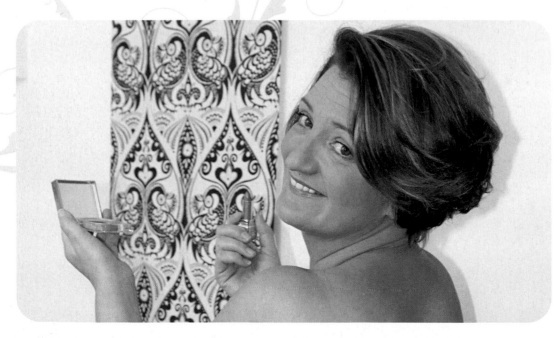

Magic pant know-how

You've heard a lot about magic pants in this book – and there's no denying they're a girl's best friend – but what you might not know is that they come in many different varieties, according to part of your body you are trying to control. Here's how to choose a pair to the suit the occasion.

HIGH-WAISTED THIGH-LENGTH PANTS
These sort you out from the waist down, smoothing thighs, bums and tums.

HIGH-LEGGED PANTS
This style pulls in your tummy and, because it is cut high in the leg, lifts your bum.

TUMMY-FLATTENER THONGS
These will enable you to avoid Visible Panty Line (VPL) syndrome while pulling in your stomach.

CINCHING BRIEFS
These briefs sit high on the leg and end around your belly button, pulling in your tummy and smoothing out your muffin top - great for creating an hourglass shape. They're also available in g-string style, so you can avoid VPL.

CONTROL DRESS
Similar to a slip, a control dress supports your breasts, pulls your tummy in and smoothes out your hips and thighs, while lifting your buttocks. The control dress basically gives you a one size smaller body reshape – perfect for that gorgeous party frock.

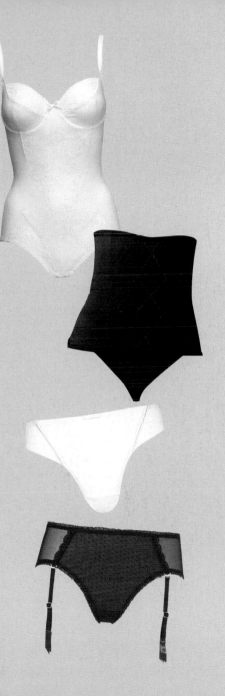

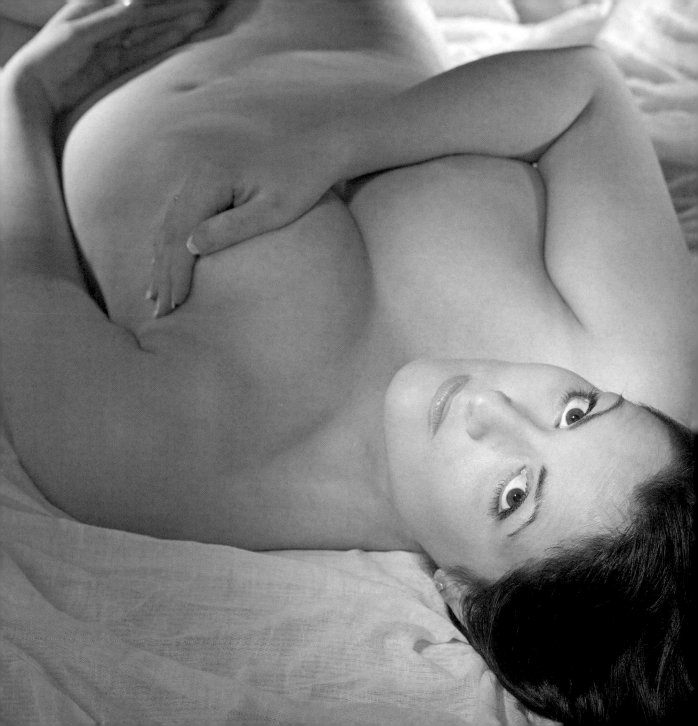

CONFIDENCE FOR A SIZE 18

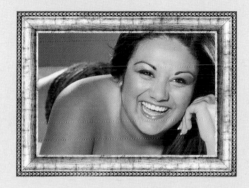

Does size really matter? Rubie Poonia certainly thought so. A PR girl by day, 25-year-old Rubie also had an evening job, working alongside the blonde and the beautiful of beachside Bournemouth. During the day, Rubie hid her voluptuous figure underneath baggy clothes, and at night, when everybody else was in their dancing gear, Rubie still insisted on hiding as much flesh as possible.

Rubie was so paranoid about her size that she even refused to get changed in front of her friends when they were getting ready for a girls' night out. Like many women, Rubie seemed only able to focus on her 'bad' points, and was missing out on her many positives.

Yet Rubie was a young, gorgeous fancy-free young woman. What's more, she really loved living it large – except when it came to her size of course. Then she felt more beached whale than beach babe.

It was our mission to show her what a wonderful body she really had, dress her for the part, and help her get out there to live life on the edge.

WHAT SHE SAW

At size 18, Rubie was only one size larger than the average British woman, but she felt that she was absolutely huge. In a line-up of women who ranged from size 16 to size 22, Rubie placed herself close to the top end, adding two dress sizes to her shape. When Rubie looked at her reflection, everything felt wrong.

'I hate the way I look,' she said. 'It's just not a good look. I feel like a complete heffalump. I don't like anything about my body. I hate my stomach, I hate my hips. I'm disgusted with myself. I look like I have let myself go, and that's because I have. I love my life, I have a fun job, but I hate my appearance.'

THE POSTER TEST

When we displayed Rubie's body on the wall of Bournemouth shopping centre she was horrified. But others weren't. We asked over one hundred people what they thought when they saw the picture of Rubie in her underwear. A third of those people guessed she was a size 14. Comments from the male audience were particularly complimentary. It's no secret that men often prefer a fuller figure, yet women constantly pressurize themselves into looking super skinny.

The right jeans for your shape

If you don't have a perfect pair of denims, then you're missing out. Every girl should have a pair that makes her feel thinner, taller and ready to party! Here's how to get it right:

- Short and wide: go for a bootleg and darkish colours. Avoid embroidery or other fussy detailing.
- Petite: buy jeans that are slightly longer than you are and team them with heels.
- Pear shape: choose boot cut or flat fit leg.
- Apple shape: go for detailed pockets that sit high and wide on your bottom. High-waisted jeans will also flatten your tummy.
- Pencil shape: look for low-rise jeans.
- Hourglass: choose dark denim, flared leg.

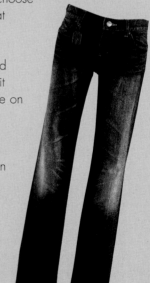

THE MAKEOVER

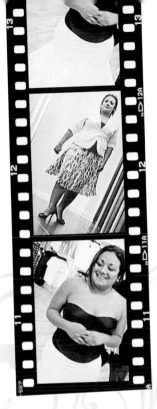

We all know that having a pair of jeans that you feel totally at home in is one of life's essentials. And what Rubie yearned for more than anything was to look good in a pair of jeans. As a size 18, she believed that this was something she could never do. But she was wrong. All sizes can wear jeans, it's just a question of choosing the right style, shape and fabric for your body – and there are a lot of different options out there (see box on p.174). For Rubie we chose high-waisted, boot cut jeans in a stretch denim to pull in her tummy. The boot cut balanced out her hips and thighs and made her legs look longer and leaner. Colour is key. Larger sizes should avoid light-coloured or distressed denim as these will make you look bigger. Instead go for dark colours, and don't wash them too often – once a week is the maximum. Avoid skinny jeans like the plague. As a finishing touch we added a pair of bright-red heels to give her some extra height.

Rubie was similarly dismissive about feminine outfits. But it was perfectly possible for her to go for a girly look. She needed to learn that she could flaunt her curves and hide the parts of her body she disliked. A gypsy-style knee-length skirt that sat on her hips showed off her slim calves and, with the correct slimming underwear, made her look curvy, not over-sized. It gave her a wonderful young and summery look. Rubie was lucky – her dark skin tone meant she was able to wear strong colours such as deep reds.

SIZE 16 SECRETS

Like a frightening number of women, Rubie had never had herself measured for a bra. In fact, she confessed that her mum bought all her underwear for her! She had been wearing a C cup since the age of 17 – but was actually an E. If you're a larger size, then it's imperative you wear the correct-sized bra and underpants. Meanwhile, let those magic knickers sort out all your lumpy bits (see p.171). An all-in-one body shaper will pull you in at least one dress size and help your clothes skim over your body.

The Rules

LARGER FIGURES

Go for

- A belt – it will draw the attention to your waist and give your lovely hourglass shape some curves.
- Colour. The right print and pattern actually make you look smaller. Remember: bigger is better.
- A darker colour on the area you wish to camouflage. A brightly-coloured top with a skirt in a darker shade will draw the attention upwards.
- V-necks or low-cut tops. They draw the eye inwards, so you're not focusing on either side of your body.
- Underwear that fits you perfectly. The right pair of knickers should hold you in, not let you hang out, while the correct sized bra will go a long way to creating an enviable cleavage.
- Accessories. They can really make an outfit and draw the attention away from problem areas. A jaunty scarf will bring the eye to your gorgeous face and away from your tum.

Avoid

- A-line tops or dresses, as they'll just add volume.
- Unstructured jackets or trousers.
- Flat shoes, unless you're combining them with an above-the-knee skirt to show off some flesh.

THE RESULT

After a session with the hair and make-up artists, Rubie was undressed to impress. 'If I'd been asked three weeks ago to pose naked, I would have said no way,' she said. But four weeks later, Rubie loved the attention she was getting. She was walking confidently into shops and trying on outfits she would never have considered before. Accessories and jewellery were a particular revelation to Rubie. 'I would never have worn a necklace,' she admitted. 'And I realize that when I do meet people they're not actually judging me. It's a relief really.'

'I've started liking myself and accepting myself again.'

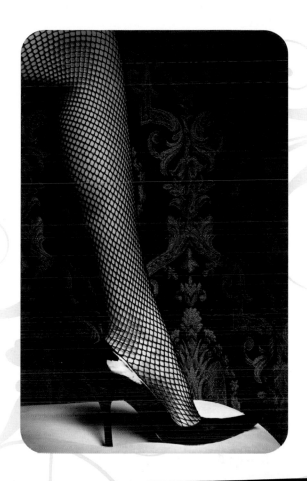

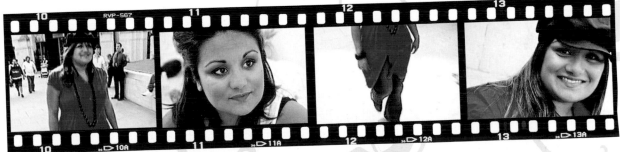

Tops

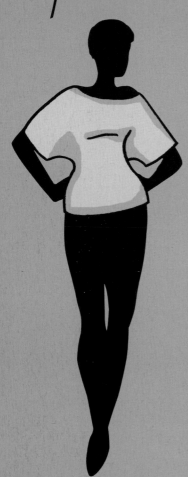

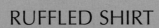

BATWING

FEATURES: wide sleeves that flare from the shoulder
GOOD FOR: pencil, pear, hourglass
BAD FOR: apple

RUFFLED SHIRT

FEATURES: soft frills
GOOD FOR: pencil, pear, hourglass
BAD FOR: apple, busty hourglass

TUNIC/SMOCK

FEATURES: flares out from above boobs, finishing at thighs
GOOD FOR: pear, pencil
BAD FOR: apple, hourglass

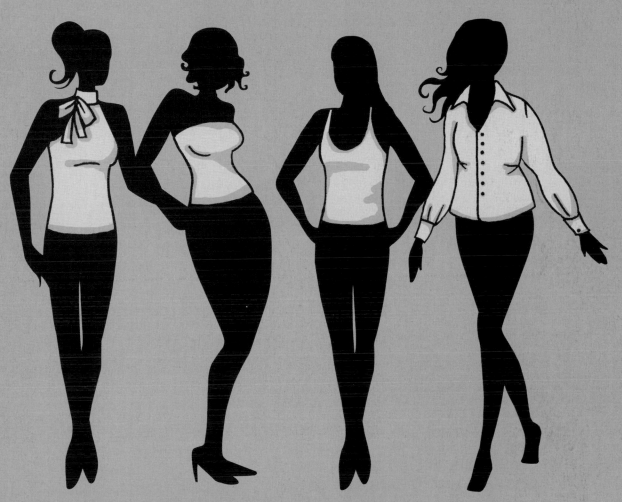

SHELL

FEATURES: sleeveless, high neckline
GOOD FOR: pencil, pear
BAD FOR: apple, hourglass

BANDEAU

FEATURES: strapless, figure-hugging
GOOD FOR: pencil, hourglass
BAD FOR: pear, apple

VEST/SLEEVELESS

FEATURES: strappy, summery
GOOD FOR: pencil, hourglass
BAD FOR: pear (unless straps are wide), apple

FITTED SHIRT

FEATURES: tailored with a nipped-in waist
GOOD FOR: all
BAD FOR: none

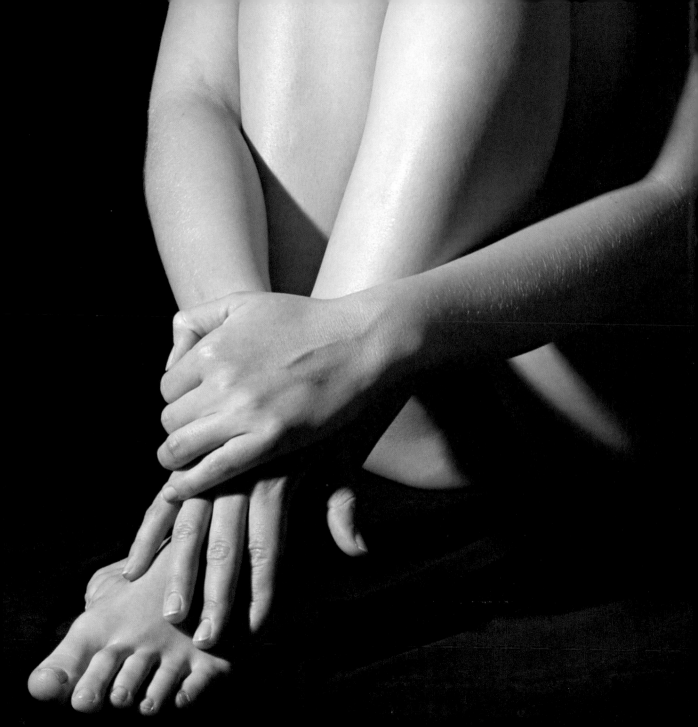

SWIMSUIT BLUES

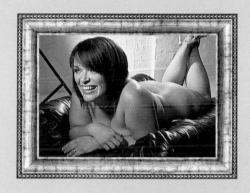

Once upon time Michelle Gower was an extrovert Essex girl who was more than happy to hit the beach in her bikini and flaunt her beautiful curves. But since having two children she had lost her spark and would no longer wear her swimsuit and take the kids for a swim. She thought that people would be disappointed if they saw her body, so she preferred to keep it hidden away.

Once full of beans and confidence, this former livewire was now more desperate housewife than devastating diva. In short, she wanted to be invisible. Her low self-esteem had begun to affect her relationship with her husband Craig. Michelle thought that her body was turning her husband off, yet he thought that there was something wrong with him! The closest Michelle came to intimacy with her husband was to wear his clothes.

Michelle had a perfect hourglass figure, the most wanted and enviable of all the body shapes. Yet the images she saw in magazines did not show her body shape, and so she thought it was wrong. We needed to get Michelle away from those mags and into something marvellous.

WHAT SHE SAW

When we brought Michelle in front of the looking glass she felt very vulnerable. She found it upsetting to see herself in her underwear and just wanted to cover up again straight away. 'Taking my clothes off in front of strangers is my worst nightmare,' she said. She hated what she referred to as her 'dinner lady arms' and couldn't see beyond her flaws to her perfect hourglass figure.

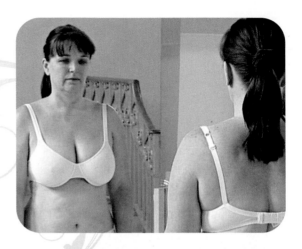

In fact, Michelle couldn't find anything to be positive about when she looked at herself naked. She hated her belly – she thought it was untoned and flabby; she disliked her boobs – she thought they were big and saggy; and she hated her thighs and the backs of her calves. 'I've just totally lost interest in myself,' she said.

Michelle's family had also noticed the changes in her and her decreased self-confidence. 'I think she's kind of given up, and she doesn't really want to be noticed anymore,' said her sister.

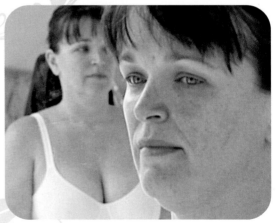

We needed to get Michelle's distorted body image back into perspective by showing her that wobbly tummies are normal, not nasty. Michelle had been so unaware of her body size that she had no idea what her stomach measurements were. She thought her belly measured about 47 inches, when it was actually a much smaller 42 inches. It was time for Michelle to be honest with herself and realize that flesh is fantastic.

🛍 THE MAKEOVER

Michelle should have been proud to show off her figure and classic sexy shape. Going in and out at all the right places, Michelle had a timeless silhouette that had been shouting out to be shown off.

As always, the underwear was the first thing that required attention. In addition to being way out on her stomach measurements, Michelle had no idea what her bra size was – a crime that 70% of women constantly commit. Once she had a bra that fitted correctly, she could see her tummy once more and was able to show off her beautiful boobs.

We chose a skirt that ended mid-calf. This was to give the illusion of endless legs that came up to a tiny waist. Michelle's new best friend, her structured jacket, topped the outfit to highlight her gorgeous shoulders while again emphasizing her small waist.

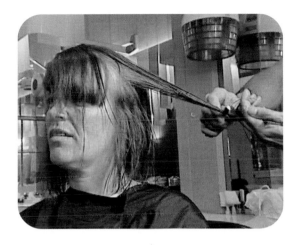

70% of women wear the wrong bra size

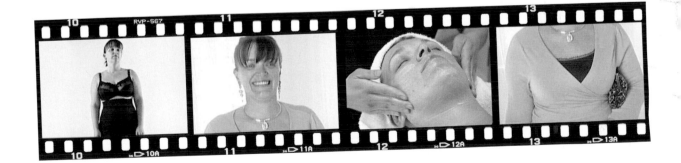

To show Michelle how to move seamlessly from day to night, we introduced her to a single outfit that worked two ways. This was a flat-fronted, wide-pleated skirt, which by day was teamed with a tummy-flattening vest top and wrap cardigan. At night, the vest and cardigan stayed, but a longer skirt gave a perfect twist for evening.

Michelle had avoided swimwear for years, but once she'd seen her body in the ruched full piece we chose for her, she understood that it was even possible to find something that would tempt her back to the beach. This style held her in and showed off her sexy back really well. A sexily-tied sarong also showed off her beautiful breasts.

Swimwear rules

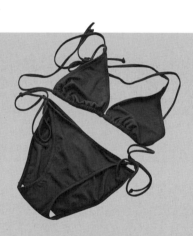

We can all look good on the beach. Here's how:

- If you have large hips and bottom, look for full pieces that ruche or gather across the tummy and hips. This will help to disguise a belly or dimpled body.

- If you're top-heavy, go for chevron stripes. These will create a more streamlined shape and flatten rounder tummies.

- If you need support up top always choose swimwear with padded or underwired bra. This will also help to create a more hourglass shape.

- If you're flat on top then a halter-neck is ideal. It gives your shoulders width and your upper body a more flattering, not flattening, shape.

- Pear shapes look great in an empire-line style full piece which draws attention away from your hips.

- Pencil shapes look great in brightly patterned swimsuits. Pencils can also choose a bandeau-style full piece that highlights their lovely, petite shoulders and creates a more classic shape.

- Plunging necklines will make anyone look taller and slimmer, so be brave and take the plunge!

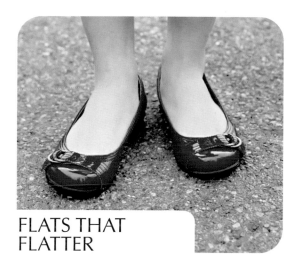

FLATS THAT FLATTER

Let's face it; it's not always practical to totter around town in heels. So if you're more likely to wear heels on a night out and flats during the day, then take a look at our guide to flats that flatter your body shape.

FLATS WITH ANKLE STRAPS
Avoid if you're petite or have thickish ankles. The ankle strap acts as an widening band and draws the attention to a part of your body you'd be better off elongating. Particularly if you're short of leg, then ankle straps will 'cut' you off, making you look more stumpy.

BALLET FLATS
Seen everywhere on the high street, these suit almost all body shapes. If you want to avoid attention being focused on your lower half, though, opt for dark or metallic colours. If you're tall or pencil shaped, then you can splash out on some brilliantly coloured ballets. If you have short, more chunky legs, only wear ballet flats with dresses that finish above the knee.

DECK SHOE
This square-toed, chunky shoe can work for all body shapes and will make your legs appear slimmer.

SANDALS
If you have short legs then avoid combining flat sandals with a hemline that finishes at calf length, as this will make you look even shorter. If you have thickish legs then avoid delicate, strappy sandals and go for something chunkier instead.

EMBROIDERED
If you're petite with small feet to match then appliquéd or embroidered shoes will help make your feet look more substantial.

FLAT BOOTS
Incredibly comfortable, but it's easy to get it wrong when it comes to the basic boot. If you're short or have thick calves and thighs, then avoid calf-length and ankle boots. Instead, opt for knee-length boots that elongate and slim the calf.

THE RESULT

With the outfits sorted, we needed to address the salon stuff. A short, sharp bob took years and pounds off Michelle's face – she looked like the gorgeous Essex girl that everyone thought had been lost forever. And what's more, Michelle braved the catwalk and the crowds for her naked photo shoot. 'I was petrified at the shoot,' she said. 'I wanted to turn round and run away. But I just kept reminding myself that this was a really important thing for me to do and I wanted to get it right. By the end I was thinking I could get used to this type of thing.'

So, in the space of eight weeks and after some serious body-loving lessons, the beach babe was finally back. 'I'm so lost for words and so tearful,' confessed husband Craig. 'I'm so proud, the proudest man in the world. She's back – I finally have my Michelle back. She even takes her clothes off in front of me now, which is something she hadn't done for a long, long time.'

> *'I just kept reminding myself that this was a really important thing for me to do and I wanted to get it right.'*

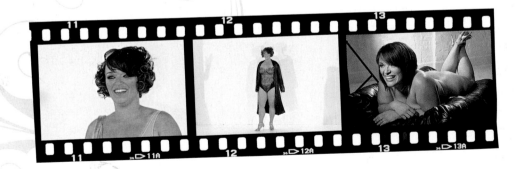

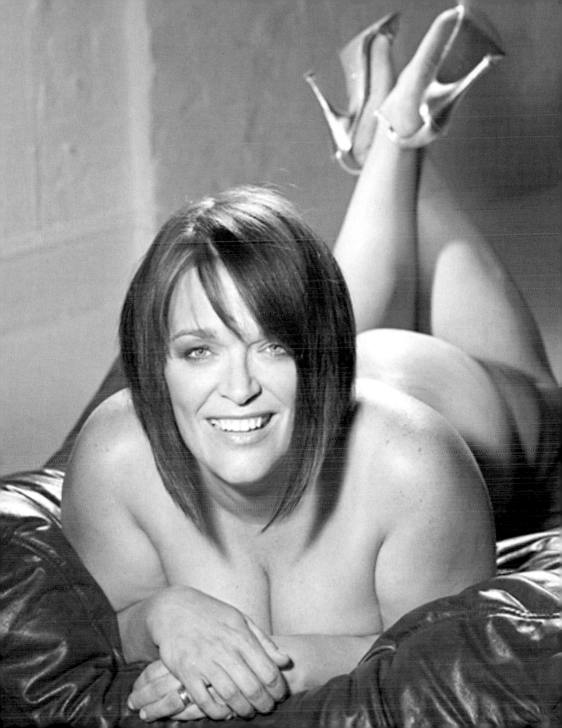

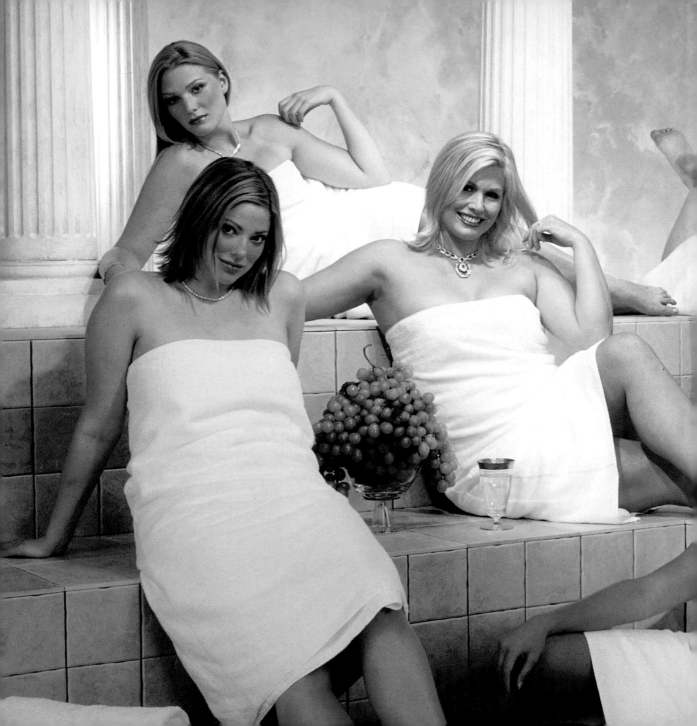

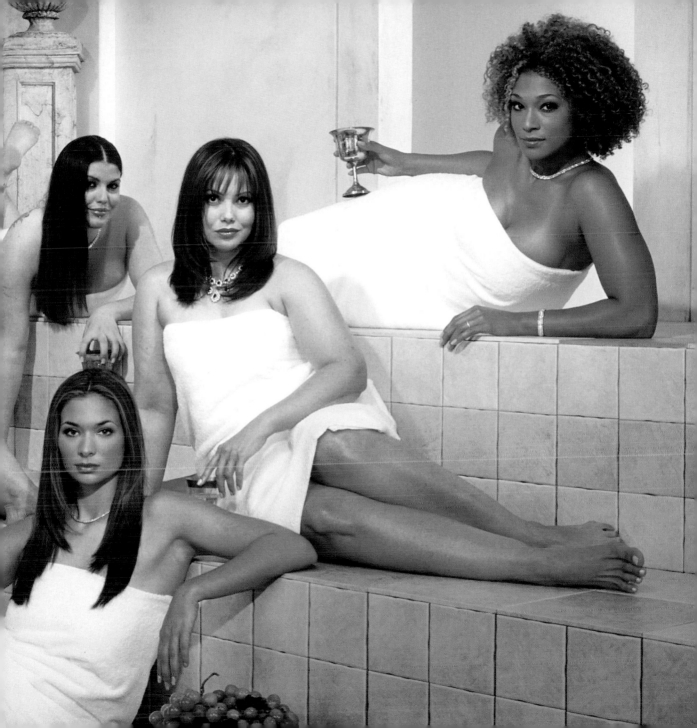

INDEX

PICTURE CREDITS

The publishers would like to thank the following organizations and photographic libraries for providing images for this book: